CONTENTS

CW00402284

Introduction.

Hello there. I still can't believe I have finished my first ever book and so I would like to say a massive thank you for supporting me, it means a lot. I hope this book helps to move you closer towards your fitness goals whilst busting some myths, giving you straight talking advice and real facts about successful fat loss. At the end of this book I have included a couple of bonuses, which are gifts from me to you to say thank you for buying this book.

So who the devil am I? Well let me introduce myself. My name is Vanessa and I have been working as a Personal Trainer for around nine years now. I haven't always been a Personal Trainer but I have always been into fitness and movement in some sort of capacity my entire life. I am a mum to my two girls called Jessica and Samantha (who are both rapidly over taking me in height). A wife to my gorgeous husband Jason who puts up with my "crazy" and gives me gentle tugs back down to earth when I get too excited and a proud owner of an adorable Yorkshire Terrier named Astro. I have lived in a town called Basingstoke, Hampshire, UK for most of my life with the odd year or two out but I have never strayed far.

I am in the fortunate position to work from home most of the time running my Online Fitness Business, guilty of being a work-a-holic, but that's because I am obsessed with helping women on their fitness journey. In the daytime it's usually just me and Astro and then the rest of the time

Mum duties call when the kids are around. Usually after dinner has been devoured we all relax and go about doing whatever families do. All seems pretty standard stuff and to anyone reading this book it sounds like I live a very idyllic life and have it all worked out. Which is, as you'd expect, why I am writing this book.

Erm no...not exactly.....

You see the thing is, I do indeed have a lovely life, but it's not been without it's challenges and I am sure there are many challenges that are on the horizon. Like most people I have experienced ups and downs. Like most women I have dealt with common issues; like having a negative body image, low self worth, battled anxiety, gone through overwhelm, winging motherhood, experiencing a lack of motivation to exercise, or over exercising to the point of obsession. I have, in the past, developed a poor relationship with food. I've drank too much alcohol, I've been too thin, I've been too fat and that's really just scratching the surface of what I have faced in the pursuit of being healthier and happier. So, I am just like you and my journey is a very familiar story to many women. I am guessing you can probably relate to a few of the above. Am I right?

I created this book because I wanted to help you. Because I don't want you to take the scenic route like I did. If I had known then what I know now, I could have saved myself a lot of time. I want you to reach a point where you finally feel happy and confident in your skin. So you can think of this book as your short cut through all that crap we read in magazines, see on social media and are sold by various companies or people. The fitness industry is worth billions and big companies depend on your insecurities to keep filling their pockets whilst you buy their products in the hope this will be the product that works for you.

Usually, by the time someone comes to me for help, they are already in a tangled web of misinformation. I then spend weeks, maybe months, helping them unpack and forget everything they thought they knew about fat loss so that we can then build some solid foundations which will actually enable them to achieve their goals the right way. And that is exactly the intention behind this book. To give you that head start and build the foundations you need to be successful in reaching your fitness goals.

These days our lives are so fast paced we want results yesterday! The thought of putting in the work can be a real turn off for women when there are so many products out there promising a bikini body in six weeks if you follow the detox, or take this pill, hence the rise of the Quick fix diet. But unfortunately these quick fix diet's only add to the problem and usually everyone who participates in them finds themselves back at square one, or in a worse off situation, once the stop it. The only way to see long lasting results is to put the work in and whilst it sounds daunting it's actually pretty simple.

Us women are far too hard on ourselves. We will often compare ourselves to our friends, but also complete strangers that we know nothing about, perceiving they look better than us or thinking they have the perfect life. Just for the record, even the most beautiful women have insecurities and nobody has life completely worked out. We are guilty of putting everyone's needs above our own. We put pressure on ourselves to be the perfect mum whilst snapping back to pre baby body; to be successful in our careers, whilst juggling motherhood or being the partner of the year. We set ourselves unrealistic expectations, chasing perfection and ultimately affecting our own body image and self esteem.

This book is based upon my findings from working with hundreds of women and drawn from my own experiences. When it comes down to it we are all very different, but at the same time we are all very similar. It's time to wipe the slate clean. Forget everything you think you know and get back to basics.

My Journey (in a nut shell)

I have led a colourful life so far. It's been full of ups and downs and sprinkled with adversity. The twists and turns in the journey of my life are something that I have come to embrace and with every shitty experience that has come along, I have tried to turn it into a positive by learning from it. Sometimes, I have had to relive that shitty experience a few times over and over until I eventually understood the lesson I was supposed to learn. It took me a while to catch on, but I got there in the end.

Our life events, our experiences and perceptions of those experiences are what shape us and our beliefs. A perfect example of this was when I was a little girl, we are talking from the age of three onwards. I was always brought up to been seen and not heard, my parents were super hot on manners. If I ever excitedly interrupted when the adults were talking, I was immediately shut down by my parents in front of our guests and told "Vanessa the adults are talking please don't interrupt". I quickly learnt impeccable manners from being told this over and over again, but ultimately the outcome from this was I went on to develop a fear of speaking my mind, or speaking up at all in case someone told me to be quiet, that my voice didn't matter. It's a small and silly example but it shows how even seemingly small things can influence us later on in life. Sure, my parents were just trying to instill good old fashioned manners, but it was at the cost of suppressing their child. Luckily for me I managed to train myself out of that habit and can now happily stand in front of a room full of people. It's also good to note that not every one will have the same interpretation of the same experience. The point being, when we bring my experience into the world of a female adult, is that it only takes a single comment about how we look from another person to affect us emotionally and cause us to dwell on that negative. If it impacts us enough it starts to manifest and chip away at our self-confidence. Slowly but surely, we start to believe what that person said to be true and then that's when negative self-talk happens and we start to nit pick at our bodies in the mirror. This is something that has happened to me many times on many different areas of life and not just around my body but also when my intellect and my personality have been commented on.

I have always been active, as a child I went to dance school from 6-12 years old, I was always outside playing and then through my late teens I joined a gym and carried my on my fitness pretty much daily. I did experience some short periods of not exercising. In my teens I seemed, like many, to be able to eat anything and everything and wake up the next day with a flat tummy. I think I was around 18, when my lifestyle was fuelled by alcohol and fast food, when I realised that I probably couldn't get away with living like that anymore, as I noticed my clothes were getting tighter. Now I had to work at it!

At the age of 18 I found the break up diet, you know the one where you can't face food when a boy breaks your heart. I don't think it was so much the boy, but more the betrayal of him cheating on me that was worse. Well a week into not being able to eat anything and I notice that I was looking really lean and I kind of secretly liked it as I'd catch my reflection in a shop window and think "oh yeah". I started getting compliments from people who noticed I'd lost weight. Bear in mind here, I was never fat in the first place, just a little extra happening. These comments from people really boosted my confidence again after the knock it experienced form that boy incident, these compliments felt good, I liked it, but it did unfortunately instilled a belief that people preferred me looking skinnier. "Click" Hello eating disorder!

Even when my appetite returned after a week or so I decided that I'd suppress it and stick to 300 calories and do two hours cardio every single day. Please never ever do that, it was a very crazy and bad idea. In two weeks I had completely changed my body and whilst on the outside I loved the attention and I seemed perfectly happy, it wasn't real happiness, in fact I had now dangerously placed all my happiness into how I looked, which was a recipe for disaster.

Sure enough this lifestyle wasn't sustainable. After a period of not eating and exercising like a loon, I rebounded BIG TIME. I went on a full on binge mode, eating and drinking whilst partying with friends, sure that was fun but again it was a little too extreme, I had a habit of doing all or nothing and never establishing a balance. Subsequently, due to me over-indulging my weight increased and I ended up being bigger than I was before I started. However, I didn't mind too much, because now I knew the secret of how to lose weight quickly. All I had to do was not eat and exercise. I knew how to cheat the system(Or so I thought) and so, I spent much of my late teens and most of my twenties, even after having my children, being stuck in this binge restrict cycle. Getting fatter then getting skinny again. Always going from one extreme to the next and never finding a balance that was sustainable. I'd like to stress that weight fluctuations are normal, a couple of pounds here and there are fine and nothing to worry about, but when it's on a such dramatic scale or a stone or two it does raise some red flags. For me those red flags were about the state of my mental health at that time. Clearly, I was struggling with self identity, I placed my self worth in how I looked and I had low self esteem. I really needed to spend some time working on me, but I just didn't know it. This extreme dieting also took a toll on my body and completely messed up my hormones causing my hair to thin and start falling out. Not ideal and an awful thing for any women to go through at such a young age, it did cause me distress. But it was the wake up call I needed to start making changes for the better.

So how on earth did I become a Personal Trainer? Well, after having my second daughter Samantha, I would have been 25, I was adamant I was getting back to my post baby body. It was harder than my first pregnancy but within two weeks I was back in my size 8 jeans. Again, absolutely crazy and in hindsight, I wish I hadn't been in such a rush to snap back and let my body recovery from the epic nine month journey it had been on. I did my usual two hour cardio stints and I ate like a sparrow. I saw results of course, but my bum completely vanished due to muscle wastage, I had no shape and it was super time consuming. One day, as I flicked through a glossy gossip magazine, I came across a photo of a lady and it made me stop and just stare at her body in complete admiration. The woman was Nell McAndrew, (if you don't know who she is Google her). This magazine had photos of her in a bikini on the beach looking incredible, relaxed and completely confident in her skin. She was lean, but not skinny, she had muscle, but didn't look manly and she looked like she had so much energy. It was as if a light switch had been flicked inside my head and just like that I decided I wanted to look like her. I wanted abs, I wanted muscle, I wanted to strut around on the beach with a hard toned body. The very next day I went to my local gym and I started to scan the room for a Personal Trainer (PT). My choice of Personal Trainer was completely impulsive and I did zero research. My method of choosing my Personal Trainer was based on how sweaty the clients looked after their session, not the most credible way of choosing your PT but I got lucky and managed to choose a trainer called Chris. I literally told Chris to make me look like Nell McAndrew. I was clueless about what getting to my goal would entail, but I can tell you now it was a real eye opener. Chris took me through a very detailed consultation and when I think about the answers I gave to his questions, I do cringe a little, but smile because I sound exactly like my clients when they come to me now. So, to cut to chase, Chris introduced me to weight training, he put me on a cardio ban and totally flipped my nutrition on it's head. I felt amazing, I saw results quickly and I loved how I could actually change my body shape by weight training. I then wondered why on earth would women spend hours doing cardio and eat like a child when they could lift weights and eat more food instead of starving themselves. So again, acting on impulse, I decided that I would help women do the same by becoming a Personal Trainer.

That was a very quick, in a nut shell, background of my journey to becoming the Personal Trainer I am today. You can see I have faced similar struggles to most women. I was not blessed with great genetics, unlike my older sister who can literally eat anything and sit on her bum yet doesn't gain any fat (we have had many jokes about we were given the wrong bodies) This meant I would also do the typical female thing and compare myself to my sister..... I digress, more about that later.

In the last eight years my passion hasn't lessened, it's just grown. I am fascinated with not just how the body works, but also the magic that brings it all together, and that is our mind set. I've learnt a great deal working with so many women over the years and from my own journey as well. For you to be successful and achieve long term sustainable fat loss, being physically fit and emotionally fit must come hand in hand and it's this which is my area of expertise and get's me fired up. Anyone can lose weight, any Personal Trainer can give you a diet plan and a training session, but to unravel the years of bad habits, to get you thinking differently and actually enjoying the process and not just the outcome, that's how you get the body you love, forever.

This book will be broken down into five main areas covering Mindset, Environment, Sleep, Exercise and Nutrition. Each of these areas will be further broken down into smaller chunks so you can pick up and put down this book at any point. Remember this book is stripping down fat loss to the core basics. If you don't have these in place, then achieving success will come with a trade off of either your physical or mental health and/ or your results will likely be short term.

Part 1. Mind set

Oh yes, the mind, an intricate and complex organ. Welcome to the human brain. Here is an interesting fact - the blood vessels in the brain are almost 100,000 miles in length. I mean, come on, how impressive is that? It literally blows my mind (pun intended).

There was a quote I read which says something along the lines of *"To master your body you must first master your mind"* . I have no idea who said this, and I may have slightly butchered this quote, but I like the message behind it because it's so true. You will never successfully reach your goals and sustain this long term if you haven't first of all conquered your thoughts. Bearing that in mind, (seriously pun not intended) this is why I have chosen the topic around mindset to be the very first section in this book to focus on.

Mindfulness is the act of being more self aware, to be in touch with your inner self, to listen to your emotions, to trust your intuition and be present in the moment. Now, I don't want to worry you at this point, thinking this book is going to be all hippy dippy and woowoo, but I do want you to keep an open mind if mindfulness is a new concept to you. Mindfulness is something that has been practiced for thousands of years and if you have been paying attention you will of noticed that in recent years it's making a comeback in a big way. People are taking to meditation and going to yoga classes or downloading apps in an attempt to achieve mindfulness and slow down the pace of their lives. However, the kind to the mindfulness I am talking about isn't about being zen and achieving enlightenment, it's about becoming more aware of your thoughts and feelings, as these are the driving forces behind our actions. Here is an easy example of what I mean. If we feel down, we can have a knee jerk reaction to comfort eat, which isn't a useful knee jerk reaction to have if your goal is fat loss. So, becoming more self aware about your triggers and your own actions is the first step in being able to stop these negative behaviours. The power of understanding how your mind works will help you massively in your fat loss and fitness journey and it is an absolutely fundamental skill to learn and nurture. It's a skill that is always developing and so, you will never reach a point where you will know everything. It's a lifetime journey of self-discovery and understanding why we do the things we do and being able to make conscious choices instead of knee jerk self destructive unconscious choices.

Up till now, every single thought you have ever had and every decision you have every made from that thought, has lead you to this very moment reading this book, good choice by the way! If you want to lose weight, then it's true that your thoughts have led you to become overweight, because it was your choice to over eat. I know, it's a bit of a harsh reality blow and it may spark a little anger or frustration when you hear this at first, but once you understand this, it does offer some clarity around why figuring out this mind set malarkey is so important in the process of reaching your fitness goals. Think of it this way, if you have the power to make the wrong choices, you also have the power to learn how to make the right choices. It all starts and stops with you.

Are you ready? We are about to go in.

Chapter 1

Self-acceptance.

Let's start with this little gem of self-acceptance. You may wonder what self- acceptance has to do with achieving a better body, because surely we are trying to move away from how we look now, to how we want to look. And, I get it, but let's flip this and look at it from another perspective.

Imagine this. You are currently 28lbs overweight and this bothers you, a lot. You're hiding in baggy clothes and avoiding social situations because you have lost your self confidence. How does this make you feel? My guess is, you would have to feel pretty low, upset and possible loathe looking in the mirror and avoid being in photos, whenever possible. Usually, we start a fitness regime when we have decided enough is enough, when we have reached a low point and found ourselves in a lot of emotional pain. The emotional pain is heart wrenching and all we want to do is run away from that feeling as fast as possible, to not feel disgusted by our reflection, to not have to worry about the clothes we wear, to not feel embarrassed or that we are being judged. This is often the very first mistake made by women when we want to change our body. We are so desperate to move as fast as possible away from the emotional pain, that two things happen. The first being, we are in a negative mind set and coming form a place of fear, negative self talk and low self-worth. The second being, we are likely to participate in what I call panic dieting, meaning we will take drastic measures in a bid to see results fast. I am talking about doing super low calorie diets or crazy detoxes. All of the above sounds really depressing doesn't it? So now, let's try to imagine the same scenario of being 28lbs overweight, but with a different perspective and approaching fat loss in a completely different way. So, this time you were feeling calmer, you looked in the mirror and wanted to make changes, but instead of feeling hatred and disgust, you were coming from a place of love for yourself. Yes, you have wobbly bits, maybe a muffin top or a tummy that hangs over your jeans, but it doesn't send you into a negative spiral. It doesn't bother in the same way, because you know that if you eat healthier and move more, today will be the last day you look like this. That every single day, from here onwards, will be a small step towards your goals and that progress is being made. So how does that make you feel now? How does that compare to the first scenario? It should feel lighter and more empowering. This is the state of mind, ultimately, you should be striving for; it offers hope that being successful in your pursuit of your goal is absolutely possible and you will even enjoy the process along the way. That is a perfect example of self-acceptance, which is the act of loving yourself as you are, whilst working towards your goals.

The next part is working out how to get into that mind set. It all sounds very nice, but if you have spent years tearing yourself apart, to think differently may be a challenge. I will be completely honest with you. It's going to take some work. Some people will be able to do this in a matter of days, whilst other will have to work harder at this, and it could take months. I guess it really depends on where your current mind set is at. Do not be discouraged if its not where you want it to be, just make this a priority to work on. I do offer some help on this, so keep reading.

Negative Self talk

The first thing to do will be to notice the negative self talk. You know what I'm talking about, the looking in the mirror, pulling yourself apart and telling yourself you're fat, telling yourself that you can't do this, or that you're ugly, or shouldn't even bother. Stop it right now and think about this. You wouldn't let your friend talk to you this way, or if she did you wouldn't be friends, so why is it OK for you to talk to yourself in such a way? Negative self talk can be a hard habit to shake off, but the idea behind it is to catch yourself in the act. Here is a little something you can try. When a negative thought about yourself creeps in, you need to bat it away and then counteract that with three positive things about you. They don't need to be physical attributes to start with, it could be something you have achieved, but make sure you think of three things to help get your mind set back into a positive place.

Practice finding positives

This one I like. It's very simple to do, although it can feel a little strange to start with, because us women are not used to giving and receiving compliments from strangers, let alone from ourselves. But, that's all going to change right? Try starting each morning looking in the mirror. If you struggle seeing your own whole reflection, then start with just your face initially, or start whilst being fully clothed and as your get more comfortable, get down to your undies or even naked! It may take a while to get comfortable just being in front of the mirror, so daily practice is essential. Now look directly at yourself…don't be shy! And say out loud three things you love about yourself. You are not allowed to say "I don't like anything", that isn't expectable and you're simply not looking hard enough and being a negative Nancy (sorry to the Nancy's reading this book). You can start with something small like your eyes, or freckles or hair and as you start to acknowledge those small positives you will start to notice more and more. You may start off saying in week one "I love my eyes, I love my smile, I love that mole on my neck", then by week four, you have progressed to "I love my legs, I love how my tummy looks different now, I love that I can wear these jeans again". My top tip would be to try saying it with a smile on your face and make sure you believe what you are saying.

Self acceptance will put your mind set in a positive place and coming from positivity rather than negativity, will make your journey towards your fitness goals easier for you. It is important that you commit to being kind to yourself and practice these two exercises daily.

Chapter 2

Make you a priority

Can I get a hell yeah! This is a big one especially for us women. Oh my goodness, the amount of times I have heard from clients, or just women in general, telling me they don't have time to sit on the toilet and do the business without being interrupted, let alone get a workout in. Now I totally get it, most of us women are wearing multiple hats and take on multiple roles. We are Mum, partner, home maker, employee, boss, friend, good citizen and we give, give, give and keep on giving, which is our very nature as women. This is amazing, but there comes a point when you have to ask yourself, at what cost? You have probably heard of the phrase **"fit your own oxygen mask first"**, the idea behind this being you must take care of yourself first before you are able to help others…and that is absolutely true. Another saying is **"You can not pour from an empty cup"**, which helps to back up what I am about to say. The emphasis here is to make sure you are placing yourself as a priority in your life, so you don't get too busy taking care for everyone else first, then leave your needs and wants at the bottom of the pile. I mean, women feel so guilty about this, but let's say this out loud. "Make **yourself** a priority in **your own life**", because if you aren't then who is?

So let's put this into real life context. A typical day may start with the alarm going off, you hit snooze, after the four snooze alarm goes off it's time to peel yourself out of bed and get the day started. You don't have time for breakfast as you need to get the kids up, make sure they are ready and have everything they need, it's go go go to make sure they get out the door on time to get them where they need to be. After you have dropped the kids off, it's then time to head off to work, traffic annoys you and you're thinking about all the things you need to do for the day. Work starts and your next eight hours are focused on making sure your boss or employees are kept happy and your customer's and client's needs are meet and deadlines are kept. Then, it's time to go pick up the kids and go home. You walk through the door with a to do list, clubs, homework, dinner, bedtime routine, catch up on housework, then eventually sit down and relax with your chosen method of self-medication, by numbing the stress with either food, alcohol or both. This only adds to the problems, because your waist line is slowly expanding and you're either too tired to do anything about it, or wonder where in the day you'd squeeze in the time to make changes. Sound familiar?

Most of us live in a highly stressed state and it can turn a once fun loving, caring and passionate women into the snappy mum, the nagging partner, the frazzled employee or boss and the whining friend. It's safe to say that they would definitely not be showing up their best self. Is any of this hitting home? Maybe your not a mum, or you don't have a partner, but that doesn't stop life being filled up with a to do list as long as your arm. If your problem is carving out time in your day to workout, or to prepare food, then there is a solution. It's a very simple solution and one you probably won't want to hear, but here it goes. You need to make time, there I said it. I told you it was simple and probably not a popular answer. You need to make some changes to the structure of your day, to delegate some chores, to relinquish the reign of control and trust that the world won't fall apart if you take 30-60 mins out of your day for you. I often find the easiest part of the day to make changes is first thing in the morning. Getting up and doing something for you, like exercising first thing, not only sets the tone for the rest of the day, it also puts you in a good mind set. Maybe you could use that extra time to prepare food for the day as well. Doing things first thing in the morning stops you from getting bogged down through the day and feeling your will power being chipped away at. Then, when it comes to the evening, you're mentally exhausted and the idea of doing a workout now seems like living hell. So, set that alarm for 30 minutes earlier, create that time you need for you. Give the kids orders to get themselves ready (if they are old enough). Trust me when I say you will feel so good afterwards you'll be bouncing off the walls and your friends and family won't know what's gotten into you. If you already workout in the morning, then you will know that feeling of accomplishment, doing something for you and having those endorphins rushing around the body. If the morning doesn't tickle your fancy then set clear boundaries designated to you getting your workout in or preparing food.

I think a common problem for us women is that we feel guilty if we decide to do something for ourselves, but we shouldn't. Why shouldn't we be a little selfish with our time? I am pretty sure nobody thinks twice when we give our time to others, but we feel like it's frowned upon to be a tiny bit self indulgent. It's time to ditch the guilt, because you are allowed to have some time for you. Give yourself permission and you will feel recharged, calmer and more focused. You may also get a little push back from friends or family when you start doing things for yourself, maybe with comments like, "going to the gym again are we?". Little digs, which they know will pull at your heart strings and make you think twice, but bat them away, because you are doing this for you, so you can show up and be better for them. They will fall in line eventually, when they realise that you're serious. (More about this later)

It's important to spend time on you, not to just exercise, because exercise can also be a kind of stress to the body if abused, but it's important to find time in your day to just be still, to be able to reflect, enjoy some music, read a book, have a bath without being interrupted and asked a million questions, to meditate, stretching or whatever your you time looks like, please if you do nothing else from this book, do this. Look for opportunities in your day where you can find time, obvious place to start first thing in the morning and last thing at night. Is there an opportunity midday to make some "you" time, so you can feel calmer? How about a walk outside during lunch, or dancing around the living room? How about after the school run? It can be as little as 5 mins, or you can take as long as you need. But, you will notice how good you feel with even just the smallest amount of you time practiced daily. I personally have about three hours of me time a day, and whilst that seems like a lot, I know it's what I need to recharge my batteries. I'm up at 5.00am and at 6.00am, I am going on camera Live to my members and then, I am just giving time to others until the school run is done. So that hour window in the morning is my quiet time for me, when the rest of the house is still and this is when I usually set my intentions for the day, do a bit of reading and journaling; filling up my cup with positive stuff. It allows me to run the day, rather than let the day run me. Once the school run is done, I have already been on the go for three hours working, so I will then either go straight to gym or take Astro for a long dog walk, or do both. This is more me time where I can get outside, or be doing something active whilst listening to music. Doing that lifts my mood, it motivates me and I feel ready to go again and get back to work. I also get my best ideas when I am out walking, feeling positive and inspired by nature. And then, finally, another part of my day will be the evening and I spend a little time reading before I go to bed if the husband is away with work. If he's home, then I don't mind so much skipping that, I know what you are thinking, get your mind out the gutter. So that's how I shape my day and honestly, if I miss a day, I can probably handle it, but miss two and I start to notice my mood dip and I start becoming lazy.

Chapter 3

Set yourself a goal

Without a goal...How will you score? Casey Nelsat

Now, you are probably thinking that this seems fairly obvious, and you'd be right, however, most people are actually not setting goals properly. Let's say for example, you get to the end of December and you are feeling fit to burst from all the yummy foods and drinking a few too many. The New Year is approaching and now you want to get fit and lose weight, like most of the population and we all make the New Years resolution that this year is going to be our healthiest yet. But, alas, with all the good intentions the vast majority fail to succeed in their New Years resolutions. And why do you think that is? It's because their goal was, how do I put this, "flakey". Let me elaborate one that for you.

Take the New Years scenario. You're feeling gross because you haven't seen a vegetable in what feels like forever, you're tired because you haven't moved much except to the dinner table and back and it's safe to say you're feeling bloated and avoiding the scales at all costs. Right now, motivation is super high and you are ready to take action, because you hate the way you feel and look at the moment. You say the magic words "This year my New Years Resolution is to lose weight and get in shape" and to give you credit you really do mean it, you're dead serious, this is happening and the world had better watch out. But, what happens next usually looks a little something like this. The first week you're on fire and doing the workouts and eating well and feeling great, week two you're still going but you're really having to battle with yourself to get the workouts in and keep on top of eating, by week three you might have skipped a couple of workouts and started rewarding yourself with "treat food", because, after all, you have been so good lately and week four those gym session are really becoming few and far between, because life is getting in the way and your food choices haven't been great because you had no other option. Eventually, the New Years' resolution becomes a distant memory and you're back to your old habits and ways. The reason why this New Years' Resolution failed and why so many other goals are not achieved is due to two missing components. The first missing component being that this goal wasn't specific enough to have any real gravity behind it. The idea to lose weight and get fit seems like a great goal, but in reality is not, because what does it really mean to lose weight and get fit? It's very vague and feels aloof and it doesn't narrow down on the nitty gritty of what you want to achieve in terms of the following. How much weight do you want to lose; one lb or one stone or five stone? How will you know when you've reached that goal? When you can walk to the top of the stairs without being breathless, when you can run 10k or when you can complete an ultra marathon? How will you do that? are you going to start running or are you going to lift weights? How will you measure you fitness levels? Being fit at what?

So instead, here is a better way to set that same goal. I am (*I am* is very important to use, because it's empowering) going to lose one stone in the next two months by getting up an hour earlier and going to the gym four times a week and starting to eat in a calorie deficit. This way of setting a goal has much more clarity around it for you, it sounds far more real and tangible now you have set a clear cut intention, given yourself a target, a time frame, structure to a routine and you have also made it realistic. Which brings me onto the final key element. Be self aware enough to know what is realistic for you. If you have never been to the gym before, then setting a goal to go six days a week may be biting off more than you can chew, so start with two or three days at first, see how you get on and then, go from there. Being realistic will help build confidence in yourself rather than setting yourself up for failure.

The second reason why goals fail is due to the lack of emotional connection to the goal. Most goals are achieved successfully when we feel passionate about something or when there are very real consequences if we don't achieve our goal. This is what we call our **BIG WHY** and the more weight behind the why, the more likely we are to follow through with our actions. Everyone's why is different because we are all motivated by different things, so you will need to discover your why. Losing weight and getting fit is a nice idea and many people want to achieve that, but if it just a nice idea that doesn't have any real deep routed emotional connection or a consequence attached to it, then it just stays as a nice idea.

To help give you a better understanding of what I mean, I shall throw in a few whys that some people have used, which are powerful and hold real weight behind them.

1. You may be a parent and currently find yourself in poor health and you would love to have the energy to play with your children and ensure to the best of your ability that you're going to be around a long time for them.
2. You decided to enter a competition or a race and are either part of a team or people are sponsoring you, you don't want to let them down.
3. You are in emotional pain and really dislike how you look and feel right now. You lack confidence and self worth. If you don't do this

now your quality of life will not improve and you risk depression and losing your self identity.

These are all very common whys and are powerful to the owners of them because they are connected to deep routed emotion and have real consequences.

Here is the good stuff. Now, the trick to feeling even stronger about these whys is to imagine that you have already achieved it. Imagine yourself running around with your kids and seeing them on their wedding day. Imagine that you triumphantly crossed the finish line of a marathon with your team and are celebrating with hugs. Imagine you are trying on a dress in a shop and feeling good about fitting into a size you never could before. Give it a try. What I want you to do now is to really get in touch with what it is you want to achieve and ask yourself why? Why do you want to achieve this? What consequences does it have if you don't achieve it? And then, how amazing will you feel once you do achieve it? Then, the next step is to sit still in a quiet room, or maybe get some uplifting music and feel that feeling of you already achieving that goal. Replay that moment over and over in your mind until that feeling becomes so strong it makes you smile. Ideally, you should commit it do this every day for 1-3 mins. Yes, you may feel a little silly, but doing this helps when you have tough days. You can draw on your why and feel that feeling of achieving it already, which will help boost you and push you forwards.

Chapter 4

Motivation and willpower

I have put motivation and willpower into one chapter, because they fit very well together. In this chapter, I am going to bust some myths around them and get you thinking about both very differently.

I am going to start on Motivation. What exactly is motivation? Well, first of al, we know it's not something we can physically see, but it's something we feel and it's very much positive energy that gives us the kick up the bum to go and take action. "I am feeling motivated" is something most people have said at some point in their lives, I know I have. So that means motivation is actually an emotion, it's a feeling and like most emotions and feelings they can come and go in waves. Nobody is ever happy or angry most of the time and therefore, no one can be motivated all of the time either. I think that's the first myth we need to debunk. I often hear people say something like "I've lost my motivation" and use that as the reason behind them not doing their workouts or sticking to their diet. It is important to understand that motivation is the stuff that get us started, it's the initial injection of enthusiasm we need to get up and join the gym, or start running, or do a healthy food shop. However, after the initial honeymoon phase, motivation does start to fade and the feeling of motivation isn't as strong any more. It can go completely and then it can come back. The problem here is that people believe that the feeling of being motivated should continue and if they don't feel motivated, then something is wrong with them and so they stop.

The saying goes **"Motivation gets you started, habits keep you going"**

During the honeymoon period, whilst your motivation is at it's highest, it would be a great idea to start building some healthy habits (I'll go into this later in more detail), but for now, think about creating a morning routine or adding more structure to your day. Create a schedule that maps out your day and devote set times for certain activities and stick to the plan. This will help to keep you going when motivation starts to subside.

Next up is willpower. As a Personal Trainer, something I hear a lot of people say is "I don't have enough willpower to do that". Like I mentioned, as with motivation, your willpower is based on how you feel and your positive energy. I like to think of willpower as a battery pack. Imagine this....Your body is fuelled by food and water, but your brain is fuelled by this big battery and just like all batteries, it needs to be recharged and topped up to keep it from running out of power. There are two things that will drain your battery a lot quicker and these are making decisions and stress. Every time you are forced to make a choice or become stressed, you drain your battery more and more. Here is a fun fact for you, it is said that the average adult make around 35,000 decisions in a single day, that sounds exhausting doesn't it? but, that tells you just how busy your brain is. Luckily for you, most of these decisions are automatically done without you even really thinking about it too much, due to automatic responses from repeating habits and routines. If you have had a very busy and stressful day, it's very likely that by the evening you feel mentally drained and flop onto your sofa. Your willpower battery has taken a battering and it's at this point when you are most likely to then say "sod it" to getting that working out in or preparing a healthy meal. It's far more likely you're so tired you will choose the easiest and quickest option, because you have what's called "decision fatigue" and the idea of sitting on the sofa and having a glass of wine is a much more appealing option and far less effort than slaving over dinner or finding the energy to go workout.

So, how do you prevent your willpower battery from draining? The answer isn't as difficult as you might think and all it takes is a little planning ahead. What you want to do is reduce the amount of decisions you ask yourself to make in a day, especially decisions around food and exercise, because these will be brand new habits and your brain isn't familiar with these yet. Start by looking at your schedule for the day and plan into your day when and what you are going to eat. If you are on the go travelling, then prepare a lunch which can travel with you. If you're out and about, make sure you keep a healthy snack in your bag. Maybe you're at the office and to avoid making poor lunch and snack decisions, you bring in a tasty home made lunch and snacks, which you can't wait to tuck into.

What about exercise? How could you remove some of the decisions around doing your workout and make that process easier? There is a lot of effort when it comes to getting your workout in, first of all we need to decide what gym clothes we are going to wear, then get dressed, then put our trainers on and finally drive to the gym, the effort of washing and drying the hair, that's without adding in life's extra complications to the mix. Again, it all comes down to planning ahead. Look at your schedule for the day and find a slot where you can dedicate that to exercise, then make that process easier on you by putting all the elements in place, so when the time comes, you're not faced with too many choices, potential barriers or resistance. If your whole day is packed, then maybe doing a workout first thing in the morning is your only choice. To set yourself up for success the night before, place your gym kit at the foot of your bed, get everything organised for the morning and have your trainers by the door. If exercising in the evening is your time, then making sure that your gym kit is in the car, so that after work you can simply get straight to the gym and do your workout before you talk yourself out of it by going home first. These are just two examples, but you get the idea, look at your daily schedule, plan ahead and remove as many potential barriers around eating the right food and getting your exercise done.

Chapter 5

Comparison

"**Comparison is the thief of joy**". Hands up, who is guilty of this? I am for sure!... not so much now, although I do have to check in with myself now and then, but definitely a few years ago. I mentioned at the start of this book how I would compare myself to my older sister, Sally, who had a size 6/8 super model body with legs up to her armpits in 'Barbie like' proportions. I am not even exaggerating! Then, there was me with my short limbs and athletic build, considering we came from the same parents we couldn't have been more different. I used to want to be like Sally so bad, but unless I was going to undergo some serious surgery, then it wasn't ever going to happen. What I am getting at is, we are all born different and we are stuck with what we've got, but it's down to us to make the most of it. Just because I wasn't blessed with supermodel genes, it didn't mean I wasn't attractive or that I don't have attributes that are pretty awesome too. It took me a long time to realise that comparing myself to my sister, or to anyone else, was just the stupidest thing to do and no good could come from it and it does nothing for your self-worth or confidence. These days, I like to be able to look at another women and appreciate how great she looks, but not let that make me feel bad about myself for not looking like that. The trick in not letting comparison affect you, comes down to self acceptance and building up your confidence within yourself. That's why doing the work on yourself daily is so important. Think of it like this, the moment you feel that you are comparing yourself to someone else, you are disrespecting yourself.   You can also use that negative comparison feeling as feedback from your brain that you need to do some work on you. It may be that you're just having an off day and simply need a bit of "you time" to fill your cup back up. But, it could be that you haven't done the work on self acceptance and losing that self negative talk, in which case, make sure you do it, everyday, until you really do believe it.

Chapter 6

Emotional Eating

This is a big one and I'm guessing the vast majority of women can relate to emotional eating in some form or another. It's all very well and good being able to stick to the diet when life is going great, but it's another story altogether when life throws us a curve ball or two. I really struggled with this in the past, having full blown binges when I was feeling stressed. In all honesty, it is something I keep checking in with, because like they say, "old habits die hard" and so, they try and creep back in if you don't keep an eye on them. The first step to mastering emotional eating is to understanding why it happens. I can best describe emotional eating as an emotional crutch, offering support and short term happiness when life is tough. So, if you find yourself feeling stressed, under pressure, anxious, depressed, upset or experiencing any negative feelings, you can instinctively turn to food for comfort. Notice that's it's always bad food, we never reach for not a salad, nobody ever craves a chicken salad when they are feeling down, it's always a nice big slab of chocolate cake.

There is actually a very real scientific reason for emotional eating, which is comforting to know, because we can feel like a women possessed when we are in the moment, unable to stop putting that slab of chocolate cake into our mouths, but at the same time knowing that we shouldn't be doing this. Let me explain it as simply as possible. When we eat something we love, like chocolate or fast food, it triggers a hit of dopamine. Dopamine is a chemical released in the brain that let's us know that what we are doing feels good and then, we store that positive feedback in our brains for when we might need it. Now, think about how many times you have eaten a bar of chocolate for example, with every single bite you are reinforcing the positive memory of how good it feels. It's likely you have gone through year upon year of positive reinforcement around a bar of chocolate. Now, imagine you are sat at home alone and experiencing emotional pain, maybe you have had an argument with your partner or something along those lines. Of course you are feeling really upset and unsettled and this is when your brain does something truly amazing by interfering. Your brain is designed to take you away from pain and uncertainty and so, in that moment when you are feeling low, the quickest and most logical route the brain can find back to your happy place would be for you to eat something that gives you that dopamine hit. Bingo, the brain knows exactly what you need … chocolate! That's when you find yourself opening the kitchen cupboards like some kind of crazy women. So, really emotional eating isn't your fault, it's your brain trying to help you out, but in reality it's just creating a bigger mess.   Whilst eating that chocolate felt good in the moment, now the guilt, shame and feeling of failure in the aftermath doesn't feel good at all leaving you feeling lower than before. This creates a vicious cycle because the brain again tells you to have more chocolate to make you happy again. We all know the best idea would be just go to bed, why do we never think of that before hand?

How do you stop emotional eating? As I said earlier, emotional eating never just goes away, instead you learn how to manage it. After years of reinforcing a rather unhealthy habit, it takes time and self awareness to avoid self sabotaging. Luckily for us, food isn't the only way to get a rush of dopamine and that is ultimately the key point for you to remember here. Whilst eating probably requires the least amount of effort, you can try a hand at the following when feel yourself getting into that state of mind.

1. Get outside and go for a walk. Being outside in nature, moving your body and fresh air can really help clear the mind and expel negative energy.
2. Do a short sharp burst of exercise. It may not be practical to get to the gym or do a full blown workout, but research has shown that as little as 5 mins of high intensity exercise is enough to help change the state of mind and boost your mood.
3. Put some music on. Make sure you put on some uplifting music, which you know elevates your mood....why not have a dance around or sing a long?
4. Speak to a friend and have a laugh. Laughter really is the best medicine, so get on the phone or go for a coffee catch up.
5. Get mindful. Try your hand at meditation or yoga, or simply have a period of time to yourself to enable you to relax your mind.
6. Sex, just throwing that one in there. Probably not practical in some situations, but you'll definitely get a hit of dopamine.

The key point here is to be aware of how you're feeling and catch yourself in the moment, just before you're about to hit the self sabotage button and implement your dopamine protocol 'go to'. It takes time to master this, so don't expect to get it straight away, but with practice it does get easier.

Chapter 7

Why I want you to fail

I do love a good quote and this one is probably one of my favourites. *"Failure doesn't mean the game is over, it means try again with experience" Len Schlesinger*. This is exactly how I see failure, but learning to view failure as a positive rather than a negative is another skill which takes time to master. The more we fail….the more we learn. The more we learn….the better equipped we are to handle the situation when it happens again. We learn far more about ourselves in the times when it didn't work out, than we do if everything is just plain sailing. The most important thing here is to not see failure as final, but as an opportunity to try again. Many women fall into the trap when dieting, that it's all got to be perfect, when in reality you just need to be better than you were before. I don't think there's much more to be said on that topic.

This picture demonstrates what success looks and feels like. It's fair to say that's a pretty accurate resemblance of my life! Would I change it?   No way, it's all valuable experience and lessons. To be honest, I am grateful for all the struggles because without them I wouldn't be who I am today without them.

SUCCESS

What people think
it looks like

What it really
looks like

Chapter 8

Stress

In todays world it's almost impossible not to come across stress unless you are a monk living in a monastery. Stress will come and go. Sometimes the magnitude of stress will be greater than other times. Knowing that stress is unavoidable, that it's within our ability to manage stress and not avoid stress, is important. Stress comes in both mental and physical forms and if stress is left to manifest in the mind and body, it can bring on serious issues. You may find burn out, anxiety, depression and other mental health issues arise, whilst on the physical side stress can lead to injury and the inability to recover from training, it lowers our immune system, causes inflammation to the body and leads to much more serious conditions effecting our heart health.

My own battles

I have always been fairly good at managing stress, I get comments all the time about how chilled out I am and they are right, I am vey much the person who views life as the glass is half full, but despite being positive most of the time, I have still had the odd bout of stress when life has gotten just too much emotionally.

It's safe to say my childhood was pretty tough and by the age of 11, I had experienced abandonment, physical abuse and death of the most important person in my life at that time, my grandmother who raised me because my parents couldn't get their act together. By the time I was 15, I experienced mental abuse, the death of my father, living in multiple homes and families from the age of 14 and being taken advantage of. This isn't the book for me to be delving into these issues, after all it's not about me it's about you, but I just wanted to give you some context as to the level of stress I experienced at such an early age and the effects this had on me. Being young, I didn't understand the gravity of these things properly, I just thought that's how life is, you power through and get on with it and I didn't want to be a burden to anyone with my problems, I didn't want to be the Debbie downer. So, I did the very British thing of showing up and putting on a brave face without even realising it. I had already dealt with a lot and I suppressed every single negative emotion I had and was hell bent on be positive and happy. This will work short term, but long term it's a recipe for disaster. People would be amazed at how "put together" I still was, how I hadn't completely gone off the rails, I mean I was no angel as a teenager, but I had a good heart. In all honesty, I look back and I do wonder. I look at my girls now and I simply can't imagine them going through such horrific things. Anyway, what do you think happened next? All the suppressed stress was manifesting away deep down and finally caught up with me when I was aged 15 and for the first time ever, I started to experience panic attacks. Back then, I had no idea what was happening to me, I thought panic attacks were people dramatically hyperventilating into paper bags, like you see in the movies. All I knew was, I was hit by an overwhelming and completely irrational sense of fear, my heart rate sped up, my breathing became quick and shallow….it was terrifying. All I wanted to do was run inside, but I couldn't because I didn't want my friends to think I was being weird, so I stood there in silence pretending to be OK as they all chatted and I tried to control my breathing. This started to happen more often and the fear got stronger, until in the end, it completely house bound me and I became too afraid to venture into open spaces. I was 16 when I realised I couldn't carry on like this and had to do something about my anxiety. It got to the point where I kept calling into work sick, because I didn't want to walk there. By that time, the stress had now come up as a physical symptom and I developed Psoriasis, which completely covered my body in scaly scabs. Psoriasis is an autoimmune illness, which is caused be inflammation in the body, in my case I was living in a highly stressed state constantly, which would trigger inflammation. To this day, nobody knows what I went through with my anxiety (well till now), because I didn't let it show. I was scared people would think I was crazy. Luckily these days, over twenty years on, mental health is spoken about freely and that's largely thanks to the great job social media has done in raising awareness about the subject. Amazingly, I managed to overcome this crippling anxiety that I had developed without seeking professional help (because I didn't know what I was experiencing had a name or that there were other people like me going through the same thing). I basically willed myself to get better, even though I was scared, I put myself into situations that terrified me and began to rationalise with myself. I came on leaps and bounds and fairly quickly the anxiety attacks became fewer and further between in under a year. If I knew then what I know now, I would have sought professional support, because even though I no longer had the anxiety attacks, I still hadn't dealt with the root cause of the issue.

Between then and now, I have gone through the usual trials and tribulations of everyday life, some phases more stressful than others, but the one thing that has helped me through all of this is having the belief that I hold the power to choose whether or not I let stress win. If I ever felt low and that life was getting on top of me, I would hit the pause button and do all the things possible to get back to me and in a good headspace again. These days, through mindfulness and being more self aware, I can manage my stress effectively and not let stress have such a grip on my mind or body again.

Stress and the effects on our body

Did you know that stress has a correlation to being overweight? In one study, it was found that women with a higher waist to hip ratio (a higher amount of tummy fat) are more likely to lead stressful lifestyles than those who didn't, linking stress as one of the factors that can lead to being overweight. As I mentioned earlier, there are two types of stress and these are mental and physical stress. Interestingly, through research it has been found that our bodies cannot distinguish the difference between the two and therefore our body will have the same response mental stress as it does to physical stress. In the modern world, the type of stress we experience today is very different to that we experienced when we were living in caves and fighting off Sabretooth Tiger, yet very little in terms of how our genetics have changed. Nowadays, our main stress would be created by the modern world like finances, work, relationships, family, holidays, moving home, lack of time and so on. Thousands of years ago, our stress would have been running away from things that posed a threat to our life, however our bodies response would remain the same in both situations. Back in the day, if we came across a threat like a Sabretooth Tiger it would immediately spark the fight or flight response in our body, which is the moment we decide whether to stay and fight or run away. To help us do this, our bodies release a sudden rush of energy, which is due to the spike of adrenaline and cortisol levels in our body, readying us to take the appropriate action. But, once the threat subsided our stress levels would return back to normal fairly quickly.

Below is an example of what happens to our body when we become stressed under the ideal circumstance. It amazes me just how clever the human body really is.

1. Your Heart Rate increases, as your body get's ready to fight or run to the threat.

2. Our body has an increase in its ability to clot. So in the event of injury, we would be able to heal a wound. (Interesting fact)

3. Our digestion shuts down. Ever noticed your appetite disappears when you are fearful? That's because your body shifts energy requirements to other areas like your limbs, lungs and heart, in case you need to run away, causing a decrease in appetite.

4. Your immune system produces more blood cells. This is a very clever response, in case you are injured and pick up an infection, as you would be better able to fight off the infection

5. Your breathing speeds up to increase oxygen to the muscles, heart and brain, so you can make a speedy get away (often not needed in modern day stressful situations, but you would have noticed your breathing speeding up).

6. Adrenaline is release into the bloodstream. The liver will release glucose and cortisol levels will raise, all giving you the energy to either fight or run from the stress.

7. Bladder and Bowel relax, due to the smooth muscle relaxing in the body. This explains why people who are anxious or scared suddenly need the number two.

8. You will start to sweat or get clammy hands. This is the body trying to eliminate toxins.

9. Muscles tense up (this can often be felt in shoulders and neck, which is a common complaint from people when feeling stressed). This is the body shifting blood flow away from skin and internal organs except for the heart and lungs.

As you can see, there is a lot that goes on in terms of how stress impacts the body. Now, under what we call "normal" circumstances, these responses should settle down quite quickly, but in today's modern world, that isn't always the case. What happens when the stress doesn't go away? What about when we find ourselves constantly worrying, on the go, not relaxing or getting angry? How does this affect our weight and ability to lose body fat?

Well, in a state of elevated and constant stress, cortisol levels remain high, this keeps you in that fight or flight state, as the brain believes the stress is still present and your body will assume you still require that rush of energy. To remain in "fight or flight" mode, your body increases blood sugar levels, by retaining sodium - ever noticed you look puffier when stressed over a prolonged period of time? Well that's why! In order to continue providing you with the demand of energy, your body will then start to crave high energy foods and these are foods which tend to be high in fats and carbohydrates. So ladies, this can also to some extent explain why we find ourselves emotional eating. However, because today's stressors are more mental than they are physical, we are not running away from anything and therefore those extra calories consumed are not being used. Instead they are deposited as fat, and usually in the tummy region. The reason why the fat is deposited in the tummy area is because it's the logical choice for the body, but it doesn't do our waistlines any favours. The excess energy we consume through food is strategically deposited as fat in the tummy, as this is close to the liver. This means that in the case of another threat, the fat stored here can be accessed easily and converted by the liver into more energy. Clever right?

This ultimately boils down to our ability to managing stress and if we don't, we can see physical stress on the body, like water retention and weight gain. The bad news is that these are just some of the effects and prolonged stress leads to much more serious issues such as mental health and heart health.

How to help manage stress

Thankfully, the awareness around stress has increased and we know that we can significantly reduce the impact of stress by implementing some really simple steps; it doesn't need to be complicated and it doesn't mean you need to become all peace and love in order to do this effectively. There are many ways to unwind and relax without the need to self medicate through alcohol and food, as doing these will just create an issue in another area of your life, that will then become a problem for you to deal with.

A couple of years ago, I went through a stressful phase of life, which carried on for months and it was causing me to be very up and down in moods, paranoid, flutters of anxiety crept in and I started to experience migraines. So, once I clocked on that actually under stress (amazing how small stress piles up without us noticing, then BAM you have that one stressor which tips the scales) I quickly made a decision to listen to my body and take action. So, I created a list of all the things I knew I enjoyed doing, that would have a positive impact on me by either calming my mind, boosting my mood or energising me. These became my "GO TO LIST" and I am telling you, it was a game changer. Now, when I feel stressed, I can get myself back into a good head space pretty quickly by doing one or sometimes more of my "GO TO LIST". These actions below are what I found works for me. Your list may be completely different.

1. Get outside and in touch with nature. I am lucky enough to live in a place which has fields, parks and greenery all around. But, just by being outside in the fresh air and having daylight on your face will help.

2. Listen to positive podcasts and read positive books. Filling your mind with positive things. I switch off the news, haven't watched that in years now and put down social media.

3. Listen to music that will lifts my mood, makes me want to dance and sing a long. Music is such a powerful tool to use.

4. Connection. Speak to a friend, give someone a call, go and grab a coffee, speak to a stranger in the shop, smiling at others when walking. We crave connection, so sitting alone in the house is not going to help.

5. Give or do something good for someone else. When the world seems down on me, it can be very easy to want to shrink inwards. Instead, when I reach out and perform an act of kindness, this makes me feel so much better.

6. Body language. I find that smiling and standing tall with my shoulders back, not only changes how I look, it changes how I feel and sometimes I'll do it with a big smile on my face.

7. Write it down. If I am feeling really overwhelmed, simply by writing down my thoughts and feelings, it helps clears my head and enables me to gain clarity.

8. Trust in the law of the universe. Nothing lasts forever and so, no matter how bad things seem to be now, change will come about.

9. Avoid dwelling on the problem and look for the solution. After all, nothing productive comes from worrying only actions.

10. Get moving the body. I could do a full on workout in the gym, or just a short five min burst, or maybe some yoga. Whatever I choose, I will be lifting my mood by realising endorphins.

11. Meditate and practice mindfulness. It can be difficult to get into meditation and it's often misunderstood. There are plenty of apps out there now that can take you through guided meditation and that's a great place to start. But, if like me you haven't completely mastered that, then just be still and learning relaxation techniques can be just as effective.

12.

Have a think about what your "Go To List" will look like, feel free to use some of my ideas if you like the sound of them. On the next page I have given you space to write down yours.

I am going to leave the mind set part here. I hope you have picked up some useful tools, maybe you had a light bulb moment, or you really resonated with parts. You may need to go back and re read this section a few times to allow it to really sink in.

My go to mood lifters

In this section make a list all the things that elevate your mood, make you smile and put you in a positive state of mind. Once you know what actions can take you there you will be able to draw up on these whenever you need them.

- ....

- ....

- ....

- ....

- ....

- ....

- ....

- ....

- ....

Part 2. Nutrition

I used to think that nutrition was the hardest part of the fitness journey, but you'll be pleased to hear that it's not. In fact it's actually the mind set stuff which is 100% the biggest hurdle. However, nutrition does come with it's own challenges, such as our relationship with food, what supplements we should take, how much we should be eating, what to eat, the best diet to follow and the list goes on. I find it fascinating that, despite nutrition being the most basic of the humans need,s we as a species, especially in developed countries, have managed to completely screw it up, making it far harder than it needs to be. The biggest reason why we struggle so much to control our appetite is the sheer amount of temptation, availability and disconnection we have with the food we are eating. Not to mention, the amount of self-medicating that's occurs around food and alcohol, or even just the unhealthy habits and ruts we have gotten ourselves into. Today, we have so much variety of delicious foods and it's right at our fingertips. I mean, we only need to walk to the shop, or drive to the supermarket, or even have our food delivered to our homes at our convenience, which is amazing. We have the technology to open our fridge and whack something in a microwave and ta'da have a meal or snack in seconds. It's a stark contrast to the situation a few hundred years ago when food was obtained through an act of killing, harvesting and also rationing, which required effort, energy expenditure and consciousness around the food we eat. The more technologically advances, the less effort is required to get food into our mouths and the bigger the disconnect between what we consume and what is actually sitting on our plates. Don't get me wrong, microwaveable meals are a life saver if you are short on time or have had a long day; the last thing you want to do is slave over a cooker for 60 mins. But, we need to be more educated and more conscious about what we are eating.

There is information overload when it comes to diet and nutrition. We are living in the digital world and you can find out the answer to just about anything on the internet. The problem here is, the world wide web isn't filtered and depending on which website you click into, you may find yourself with two very different answers on the same subject and both may have compelling information to support their answers. This is what happens when people "Google" nutrition. You could probably find 10 reasons why you should avoid avocados, because they are bad for your health and then, find 10 reasons why avocados are the best thing ever and you should eat them every day! There is a lot of conflicting and mis-guiding information out there, leaving women confused and a little overwhelmed, which causes analysis paralysis, or we end up diet hopping from one diet to the next in the hope that the next diet is going to work for us.

Nutrition is a big deal, so it needed its' own section. I am going to break it down and make it super easy for you to understand nutrition. I promise you that after reading this, you will realise it's not that complicated and you may even think it's a little dull and unsexy, because it's too simple. However, once you understand the basics it, removes the stress around nutrition.

Chapter 9

Calories and our body

Calories are little tiny creatures that come into your wardrobe at night and sew your clothes tighter. Only kidding, actually a calorie simply put is a unit of energy. One calorie is equal to one unit of energy and our body then uses that energy. A quick example of this is a sandwich containing 400 calories is equal to 400 units of energy. Everybody has a set number of daily calories/ energy units that their body needs for very basic functioning like, breathing, heart function, blinking, the digestive system etc and this is called your Basal Metabolic Rate or BMR for short. You then factor in your activity levels, which burns additional calories/ energy and that gives you the total number of calories you would need to consume daily. With me so far? The UK government has set calorie guidelines for the average man and women with an average intake of 2500 for a male and 2000 for a female, well that's what you read on most cereal boxes these days. The key thing to remember is that this is the *average* and people's actual needs will vary. The more accurate number of daily calories you require will depend on each individual and be determined by a number of factors like gender, age, height, weight and activity. Generally speaking, if you're a well built male with huge biceps and a six pack, who is in their twenties and super active, then you will require a lot more calories than a lady who is petite with little muscle mass, who is in her fifties and does yoga two times a week.

THE 3 LAWS

Here are some very basic facts that are the laws of nutrition that govern everything.

1. 1 lb of fat is equal to 3500 calories

2. To lose fat you must be in a calories deficit (expend more energy than is consumed)

3. To gain fat you must be in a calories surplus (consume more energy than you expend)

There you have it, the three laws about calories, which if followed, will get you where you need to be. When it's broken down like that, you realise just how simple it really is and yet, the vast majority of us find it the hardest thing to master and find ourselves having a bad relationship with food and our body.

How many calories?

First things first, just how many calories should you be eating? This is where it get's a little tricky and I don't want to over complicate this, but it definitely needs to be addressed. I mentioned at the start of this chapter that everyone is different in terms of our body shape, muscle mass, activity levels and also how years of dieting have affected our bodies. It would be irresponsible of me give you the tools to work that out without offering further guidance and helping you on a more personal and one to one level. If you really want to find out how many calories you should be eating, there are various calculators online which will work it out for you. But, just giving you a heads up, that these are not an exact science and they often end up calculating either very low or very high calories, they are effectively an educated best guest. I have always found the best way to work out your calories consumption is by simply tracking and adjusting. Track your nutrition via a Food Diary and body statistics (weight, body circumference measurements and how clothes fit). Here are the steps to break this down:-

1. **Weigh yourself first thing in the morning after you have had a morning wee and before you eat or drink anything.** *Doing this first thing allows you to capture your truest weight. You see, whilst we sleep our bodies think of sleep as pressing the reset button for the body. Hormone levels, digestive system and nervous system are rested. Plus, your body uses this time to repair muscles and recover the body.*

2. **Then, spend a week eating as you normally would and record your food and drink intake in as much detail as possible either on a note pad or in an app. At the end of the week, tally up the total amount of calories you consumed and divide that number by 7 to give you the average daily intake.** *I like to use an app called myfitnesspal, because it's more accurate and it gives you the calorie intake for each food rather*

than you having to find this out yourself, but it's up to you.

3. **Finally the morning of day eight, wake up and weigh yourself again and see what the results on the scales are. You will have had one of three outcomes.**
   a. Your weight has stayed the same. Meaning, you have found your maintenance calories.

   b. Your weight has gone up. Meaning you have found your calories leading to gaining fat.

   c. Your weight has gone down. Meaning, you have found your calories for fat loss.

What now? If you found that you are in a calorie deficit and you have lost weight, then if that's your goal, you don't need to do anything and continue with that amount of calories until the results stop. Then you tweak and drop the calories by 50-100 a day to encourage more results.

If you found yourself in maintenance and your weight didn't move, then you will need to drop calories by 100 a day to encourage fat loss.

If you gained weight, then dropping calories by 250 a day would be enough to encourage fat loss.

That really is the most simple and real way of knowing what your calories intake should be. You just need to be consistent with the tracking of your calories.

Myth Buster. Less isn't always better. I want to drive home this message to women, because it's a horrible belief that women need to shake off…. it simply isn't true. Yes, we must be in a calories deficit to lose weight, but many women take it to the extreme, which can cause a couple of issues, which I am going to highlight here. The yo-yo dieting hamster wheel normally goes a little something like this. A women, let's call her Sandra, starts a diet and she sees amazing results within a the relatively short space of time, say three weeks. Usually, when we see such dramatic results quickly, it's because the diet has been extremely restrictive and we have dramatically slashed the number of calories consumed each day. Let's say Sandra was eating 2,000 calories before she started her diet and now eats 1,200 a day instead. This is a whooping 800 calorie drop and is almost half of the amount of food she was consuming before the diet started. In this situation, most women will be OK for a couple of weeks as they are feeling motivated, but as the days go by, it becomes harder to stick to such a low calorie intake, as it's too restrictive in food choices. Her food portions are too small and it has been a huge lifestyle adjustment, too fast to get used to. Subsequently, Sandra slips up on her diet, feels she has failed, finding it to hard to maintain long term, causing her to rebound and fall back into old habits. Sound familiar to you?

When it comes to eating less calories in order to lose fat, you need to be sensible about how far into the calories deficit you go. Eat too few calories and not only do you risk the above scenario you also massively reduce the amount of vital vitamins and minerals needed to keep you healthy and happy. Remember me saying that I messed up my hormones? Well that was due to my excessive yo-yo dieting, my lovely thick curly hair went thin and started to fall out, which isn't fun for anyone, let alone a female in her late teens and early twenties, and that was all due to me disrupting my hormonal balance, due to under eating causing stress on my body. The lesson I learned was, you can not cheat the system and get to your goal quicker, there is always a trade off made when we take short cuts and it's usually to our health and wellbeing, it's definitely not worth it. If you are tired of this start stop dieting behaviour, then you need to develop be willing to invest some time in order to see sustainable long term results. The sweet spot will be losing weight at around 0.5 – 1lb a week. It's not a lot I know, but that drop in weight consistently compounded over 14 weeks is much better than losing 14lb in 4 weeks only to gain it back and start again.

Chapter 10

What we should know about food.

That's calories out of the way….the next thing you need to know about is the type of foods you're eating and the role each type plays. I am going to keep this short and sweet. Your food is broken down into three main categories;

Proteins, Fats and Carbohydrates. Each of these food groups has a role to play when it comes to nutrition.

Protein has been getting a lot of attention recently and there has definitely been an increased awareness around the benefits of protein in relation to our fitness, which is a great thing. Your body is made from protein. Our muscles, skin, hair nails and organs are all protein. Our body can't produce protein, so we need to get this from the food we consume. Food sources like poultry, meats, eggs, fish and diary have the highest levels of protein but it can also be found in soy, nuts, beans and vegetables. I'm not getting into the debate of whether you should eat meat or not, that's a personal choice. However, just so you know, you can absolutely get enough protein eating a vegetarian or vegan diet and it doesn't put you at a disadvantage, it just takes a little more planning and thought around what you eat. Over the years coaching women, a common worry of theirs is that eating protein will make them bulky or look like a man. Honestly, hand on heart it wont, this is a myth due to its' association as the food of bodybuilders. I have been weight training and eating a high protein based diet for the last 10 years and I have yet to be told I look manly. In fact, if you don't eat protein you're going to struggle to maintain a tight toned body.

Three reasons why you should be eating protein

1. It helps build, repair and recover muscle from training.
2. It helps support and maintain muscle mass, which increases metabolism.

3. It helps to keep you fuller for longer.

You are probably wondering how much protein you should eat? Well that does depend on the person, their goals and personal preferences. But, to get you started, try having a good serving of protein at your three main meals of the day, so Breakfast, Lunch and Dinner, this will get you well on the way. FYI a serving would be a medium sized chicken breast or to be more precise 25 gram of protein or the thickness and size of the palm of your hand. When you get comfortable with this, or if you wanted to increase your intake, you can then top this up with protein snacks.

Fat is another misunderstood macronutrient food group. In the 80's and 90's low fat diets were really popular and still are today. Food Companies and Slimming Clubs were big on promoting low fat diets and they still do today. The reason why low fat diets became popular was because by limiting an entire food group, especially fat, it will automatically lower the overall calories consumed on a daily basis. Part of the reason fat was ditched is the fact it has a higher amount of calories per gram compared to proteins and carbohydrates. A little fact here: Fat has nine calories per gram, whilst protein and carbs both have four calories per gram. By having a low fat diet, you would see a big drop in calories and the result would be weight loss. However, as always, there is a trade off when you take this to the extreme and that is women miss out on essential fatty acids, which are important, because your body cannot produce them on their own. If you are deficient in Essential Fatty Acids, then you can experience skin conditions, alopecia and mental cognition. Foods such as oily fish and nuts are fantastic sources of Essential Fatty Acids.

But not all fats are equal, so you do need to watch your intake. The rule of thumb to follow would be to eat mainly naturally occurring fat that you would find in foods like nuts, fruits, oily fish and some plants. Go easy on the red meat, animal skin and diary. Avoid as much as possible the type of fat you would find in processed foods, as these are trans fats and do have links to poor health conditions.

Carbohydrates are the third food group we are going to talk about. Carbs are the bodies preferred source of energy and can be found in many foods like fruits and vegetables, root vegetables, grains, beans, honey and also breads, oats, cakes and yummy food like that.

In the 00's celebrities seemed to favour the low carb diets such at the Atkins, Keto and Paleo diet and whilst they all had different rules, these diets followed a basic principle of consuming no or very low carbs. Again, the elimination or a big reduction of carbs meant that a whole food group was missing and of course that would results in a drop of calories automatically and women would lose weight and fast! You see, the thing about low carb diets is that during the first couple of weeks you will see a huge drop in weight when you step on the scale. Unfortunately, the majority of that weight loss is superficially and not actually fat. Let me explain how that works. For every gram of carb you eat your body will take on 2.7 grams of water on average. So if you are a big carb eater, then go on a no carb diet and it will impact the scales dramatically. The down side to a no carb diet is that it's very restrictive and most people do not last longer than 2-6 weeks before they break and usually rebound. The rebound being particularly bad and resulting in binging on all the foods they have missed out on and not had in the past few weeks. A myth I am going to bust here is that carbohydrates make you fat. They don't. If you ate nothing but carbs and went over your calorie intake, then yes, you would gain fat, but carbohydrates alone are not the problem. The low carb trend has sparked a fear into women around carbs, but if incorporated into a well balanced diet, you can eat carbs and not have any problems.

Chapter 11

What is the best diet?

I think we can all agree that there are a ton of diets to choose from. I should know, as I feel like I have tried most of them back in the day, before I knew any better. All of which failed me, made me miserable, or maybe I failed them? Whatever ... the point is, they didn't work out and the reason for that is because they just weren't the right diet for me.

Before I get into what is the best diet for you, I think we should talk about fad diets and gimmicks first. You know when they say, "If it sounds too good to be true then it usually is", well that's exactly how I see fad diets or gimmicks. Products that promise quick results usually have a trade off somewhere and it's either going to be enjoyment, sacrificing lifestyle or health and wellness. I'm talking about products like carb blockers, fat burners, detox teas and coffees. Yes, they will work short term, but the trade off isn't worth it, not to mention that you can spend a small fortune on all sorts on diet gimmicks. You'd be much better off physically and have a healthier bank balance by reading this book and investing your time into learning what really works. I would describe fad diets and gimmicks as methods or products that promise amazing weight loss results in a relatively short space of time. You have seen them sitting on the shelves in the health food shops, which in itself is ironic, because they are not good for your health at all. In most cases, these are nothing more than cleverly packaged laxatives, appetite suppressants or claim to block the absorption or carbs. Yes, you may lose weight, but is it good for your health? Probably not. I will try my best not to get ranty, but this is my biggest gripe when it comes to the Health and Fitness Industry. Big companies taking advantage of women's insecurities (how we look) and selling them the dream through a quick fix gimmick. Let's not forget that it's a big business in the female weight loss market, that's how they can afford to pay celebrities big endorsements to advertise their products. I shall leave that there before I get myself into trouble!

The truth is that all diets work! All diets work, because they all have the same one thing in common and that is a calorie deficit. So what is the best diet? Well in order to find that out, you need to take into consideration the enjoyment, compatibility and sustainability of the diet you choose. Ask yourself if you enjoy eating this way? Now, I don't know about you, but I am a foodie, I love my food, I don't like people picking food from my plate and if I share my food with you, then you are special! Food is meant to be enjoyed, you don't want to be stuck on a diet eating boring and bland tasting food that turns you off. Let's face it, if you don't enjoy your food, you are less likely going to stick to it. The next thing you need to look at is the compatibility of the diet to your lifestyle. If you're cooking two or three different meals for the family or your diet is an inconvenience to your lifestyle, then it will just become frustrating burden. Finally, the last thing you need to think about is, can you see yourself eating this way in 12 or even six months' time from now? If you can't, then this probably isn't going to be the most suitable diet for you. I mean seriously, who in their right mind will still be eating cabbage soup after two weeks? In case you are wondering, I am a stable three meals a day kind of girl, with a couple of snacks a day.

Whilst we are on the topic of the best diet, let's also look at what are the best types of foods to eat. In my world there is no such thing as good or bad foods. I don't believe in giving food labels, as it can develop a poor relationship with food. If you label a chocolate bar as a so called *bad food* and one day you're eating a chocolate bar, how on earth are you supposed to enjoy that chocolate bar without the pangs of guilt? You won't, because you would have associated it with being bad. So, instead of labelling food good or bad, I like ask myself if what I am eating will nourish my body. By understanding that some foods have more nutritional benefits than others, it gives me the power to make a conscious choice about eating that chocolate bar. If I eat it that's fine, I'd just make sure that the rest of my day I ate more nutritionally beneficial food to balance it out. If we want to lead a healthier and fitter lifestyle....I am presuming that you do if you are reading this....then we need to eat a diet mainly consisting of nutritionally beneficial food. I just want to make the link here very briefly back to calories. Our body does not discriminate between good calories or bad calories, it just knows that food is coming in and that equals calories are coming in which is energy for the body. So, whether it's 100 calories coming from an apple, or 100 calories in the form of a chocolate biscuit, the body doesn't recognise the difference and will use the energy from both to fuel it. You can still over eat and gain fat on a healthy, clean eating diet by consuming foods like nuts, granola, avocados, oily fish, oils, red meats, eggs, butter, dried fruits, juices and such. They are all at the end of the day a form of energy. You could even gain weight by eating nothing but broccoli too, but that would be a whole lot of broccoli!

The important thing to remember here is that, as long as you are eating 80% of your daily calories intake from nutritionally beneficial foods, then allowing 20% to come from a little of what you fancy isn't the end of the world. This helps to maintain a balanced diet and also keep you sane and not feeling like you are being restricted or missing out.

Chapter 12

Supplements

A question I am asked a lot is on the topic of supplements and what they should be taking, so I thought this needed to be covered briefly. So, first of all, what are supplements? When we talk about supplements, we are referring to vitamins and minerals mainly, but other things that fall under this category could be Whey protein powder, Protein bars and Fat burners. There are other supplements, but we don't need to go there. The word supplement means to add in order to complete or to enhance. And that's exactly how I view supplementation. In my humble opinion, supplements should only be introduced once you have all your basic boxes ticked, because most of what we need as humans can be consumed through good nutrition and managed by getting enough sunlight, adequate sleep and keeping stress levels in check. If you can tick these boxes, or at least tried to do your best, then it's time to introduce supplements, depending on what you deem yourself to be lacking in, or need help supporting.

I have a fairly good handle on my basics. I eat a wide variety of colourful vegetables and fruit, so I'm getting a decent amount of vitamins in. I get outside in the fresh air daily whilst I am walking Astro (my dog), which means I am absorbing sunlight and get enough vitamin D. I exercise regularly, get enough sleep and manage my stress pretty effectively. I don't actually take any vitamins as of writing this, just because I can't be bothered, but occasionally I might and if I do, it's more to really cover the bases and because I have spare cash to play with. Supplements such at Vit C, fish oil and a good multi vitamin are my essentials

Next up, let's talk protein supplements. Protein supplements like protein shakes and protein bars, I approach much like I do vitamins, the best idea would be to make sure you have consumed most of your protein requirements via actual food. However, if you are struggling to eat enough protein, or fancy upping protein levels a touch by using supplements, then go ahead by all means. Remember that protein will not make you bulky and it will help keep you fuller for longer.

Chapter 13

Alcohol

This is a juicy subject to be digging into. Personally, these days, I am not a big drinker and it's not because I am against it, but purely down to the lifestyle I live...there is just very little place for it. If I am trying to be the healthiest version of me, feel good and have good quality sleep, then I can't do that if I am drinking on a regular basis, as for me alcohol disrupts all of that. After a night on the booze my immune system takes a battering, my sleep is shocking, I feel groggy the next day and all I want to eat the next day is a bacon sandwich followed by anything carby and salty that I can fit into my mouth. Not ideal. I probably have a few glasses a handful of times in the year, but I would have thought it through to see if the trade off was worth it. This is a stark contrast from the person I used to be. I used to be the party girl who loved a drink, not so much for the taste, but more for the feeling of losing inhibitions and gaining confidence. I would drink five nights a week as a carefree adult with no kids or responsibilities, even after kids, a good night of binge drinking and dancing was the perfect release to blow off some steam. So I get it, I have been there.

Many women I coach do struggle with alcohol consumption, not because they are alcoholics but usually around social situations, either because it's now just habitual, expected of them or because they feel more relaxed after one or two drinks and we know how easily that can quickly become six or seven drinks and a dirty kebab later. Some women find a glass of wine after work helps to switch off the brain and this is perfectly acceptable until you realise you can't switch off without it. I often find women are desperate to lose body fat, but they are equally not willing to change their drinking habits to achieve it, it really comes down to alcohol acting as a emotional crutch to either numb the stress or give you confidence to be yourself in social situations. I am not saying you shouldn't drink, I believe you can absolutely drink and achieve fat loss once you know how, I am saying make sure you know how to achieve these states of mind without needing to resort to alcohol to do that for you. If you are stressed, then how else could you unwind? If you need a confidence boost, then the more you put yourself in that social situation without alcohol, the more it will help to overcome that.

Another point around alcohol is that these are empty calories. Alcohol doesn't fit into any macronutrient bracket. It's not a fat, a carbs nor a protein. In fact alcohol sit's on it's own proudly. Here is a fact for you: We know that carbohydrates and protein both have four calories per gram and fats have nine calories per gram, alcohol has seven calories per gram. When you understand this and then start doing the math on a bottle of wine, or a night out with the girls, you realise that actually the impact from alcohol can be significant.

When it comes to managing alcohol and fat loss, you than have two choices; Option one: You will go over your calories intake for the day by drinking and sacrifice your progress or Option two: You drink, but deduct those calories from your food intake either that day or the following day or spread across one, two or three days and maintain a calories deficit, so you keep moving towards your goals. Option two is a great way to combine alcohol whilst you still move towards your goals, but it doesn't mean you can abuse the system and end up having a liquid diet....remember everything in moderation. If you stick to the 80/20 and have 80% of your calorie coming from nutritious sources, then you can work in a little of what you

Part 3

Set yourself up for success

In order to give yourself the best possible chance of success, make sure you have set yourself up for success. Setting yourself up for success will make the process much easier or at least a smoother and less bumpy ride. We are all products of our environment, our lifestyle, the people we surround ourselves with, where we work, how we work and the habits we have formed. If you want to change, then it makes sense that changes need to be made in these areas of your life that are not serving you or moving you closer towards your goal. Making change is hard, because we have become so accustomed and comfortable with how things are done, so don't be hard on yourself if it doesn't all magically click into place as change takes time, persistence and patience.

"Change is hard at first, messy in the middle and gorgeous in the end" Robin Shar

Chapter 14

Environment

Our environment constitutes of all the things we have around us. I can't go into every single detail in your life, so instead I'll put them into three main areas, which are; your home environment, your work environment and your training environment. You can then assess it yourself and see what changes you can implement.

Home

At home we like to make our life comfortable and of course why wouldn't we? It's the one place we can truly relax and unwind without anyone judging us. If I want to sit in my husband's baggy tracksuit bottoms and hoodie and eat pizza, then I can. But, if we have goals, like losing a little bit of fluff around the waistline, then we have to be realistic about the behaviours we endorse at home and hold ourselves accountable. Just because no one is there watching us, it doesn't mean it didn't happen.

Remove temptation

I shall kick off the environment section by talking about triggers; more specially triggers around food. I am going to use myself as an example here. It's no secret that I am a self confessed chocoholic, I love the stuff and eat it every day, yes that's right, every day, "My name is Vanessa, I am 37 years old and I am a chocoholic", there I said it! The good thing is, I am also self-aware enough to know that I seem to have a faulty "off" switch when it comes to eating sweet foods and so, chocolate can cause me a bit of an issue if I am not mindful about it. But, what triggers these chocolate cravings? For me it's the evenings when I am bored and I get twitching hands. During the day I am busy, going about my work life and mum duties, so I am on the go all the time. But, once I have made dinner and the evening start's, I get fidgety and bored and it's that boredom, or need to do something, that makes me stand up, walk straight into my kitchen and start opening and closing the cupboards in the hope that some food will magically appear that is calorie free and tastes amazing. Note, I am not hungry it's purely for something to do. This is a pretty common behavioural trait in women. Now, if I was having such an evening in the past and those kitchen cupboards were stocked with chocolate, then I would have got myself into a pickle and devoured everything. However, I am happy to report that these days this isn't a problem and that's because I did two things. The first was, I decided to not keep chocolate in the house. This could be the same for anyone who wanted to not drink a glass of wine every night, just don't keep it in. Doing this removes the temptation and it's out of the equation. Going back a few chapters, I wrote about willpower and how it was being chipped away at throughout the day, I would be absolutely crazy to think that my willpower would hold out every single time, so I don't even give myself a chance to put myself in that position. The second thing I did, was to understand the trigger, the need for chocolate. Was I bored? Was I uncomfortable with having nothing to do? Was this just a bad habit? Was I stressed? I would reflect on how I was feeling and try and work it out from there. Understanding why is going to help, because you can then take action. If I was bored, I could find something to do. If I was stressed, then I'd need to unwind.

When I talk to women about clearing out their kitchen cupboards, I do get a mixed reaction. Some women are more than willing to give their kitchen cupboards a healthy makeover, whilst others are more reluctant as it robs them of their security blanket and emotional crutch, should the need arise.

A good idea would be to stock up on equally tasty, but healthier alternatives, like blueberries, dark chocolate, Greek yogurt and popcorn. That way, you still continue the habit and satisfy a need, but you're not sabotaging your progress and you're kind of tricking the brain. "But what about my kids, as they have to have their treats?". That's often another objection I get when I bring up a good kitchen cleanse. My comeback to this one has two parts and the first part being this. Do they have to have a treat cupboard? Is that a healthy example to set? My suggestion is, if they want sweet treats, why not walk to the local shop and buy them as and when? At least that way, they are getting some exercise at the same time. Or a nifty little trick I learnt, was to simply buy the stuff that I didn't like. This meant we would have Jammy Dodgers in our house instead of chocolate bars, because Jammy Dodgers just don't float my boat.

Morning Routine

I am a huge a huge fan of having a morning routine, for me it sets the tone for the rest of the day and is something I have done for the last five to six years and I have been consistent with it 90% of the time. Nobody wants to be that person who wakes up with the alarm screeching, pressing snooze multiple times until you eventually drag your butt out of bed and then it's just go Go GO! ... Get the kids ready, get you ready, skipping breakfast, because you have no time and you rush out the door feeling chaotic and your stress levels are already through the roof. If that's how you start your day, then the likelihood is, that's how the rest of the day will pan out too. By having a solid morning routine, you can wake up, set your intentions for the day and it allows you to run the day and not let the day run you. Sounds good doesn't it?

Here is what my typical weekday morning routine looks like just to give you some kind of idea. I am not suggesting you get up as early as me or that your routine needs to look anything like mine, it doesn't. My morning routine started out very simple from having a cup of coffee in peace and quiet, collecting my thoughts whilst everyone is asleep. Now it's slightly different, as I added things over the years.

Time	Action
05.00 – 05.20	– Alarm goes off. I get up and get myself dressed, I have already laid my clothes out the night before so I know what I am wearing. I go down stairs and I make myself a herbal tea.
05.30 – 06.00	I write in my journal, practice gratitude and set my intentions/to do list for the day. All whilst the house is quiet and everyone else is asleep and I sip my tea and fill my head with positive thoughts. Quick check social media. A girl need to keep up to date with what's happening in the world and have a good nose.
06.00 – 06.30	– It's work time. I broadcast live to my V.Fit Online Bootcamp members and do a sweaty 20 min HIIT workout. It's actually an awesome way to start the day.
06.30 – 07.00	I upload my workout videos to various social media platforms/ catch up on emails/ and other work bits.
07.00 – 07.30	shower and get dressed
07.30 – 08.00	Eat Breakfast and get out the door for the school run at 8am

A few things to take note of here;-

1. I have woken up and already laid my workouts clothes ready for the morning the night before. This means, when I wake up, I don't need to make any decisions and I can just do it without thinking. If you want to make the gym part of your morning routine that is an excellent tip. Doing this helps when we get those off days, we all get them, we wake up and just don't feel like going to the gym. But, because our workout clothes are there neatly laid out and ready, it is far more likely we will go because it will prompt us to take action.

2. I start my day calmly, caffeine isn't the first thing I drink and instead I will drink a herbal tea. This helps to not spike cortisol level too high and it's kinder to the gut

3. I spend some time on being quiet, no TV, no technology, no one else, just me and my thoughts as I write in my journal.

4. I set my intentions for the day; I write down a list of things I want to accomplish for the day. It could be that I just want to get a workout done, or to get a certain number of steps in, or eat five portions of veg or remember to call a friend. But, what my intensions are, I write them down, so I am super clear about them.

5. I get a workout in early. Doing something that raises my heart rate first thing in the morning not only ticks off the list a workout, but also puts me in a positive headspace and I feel energised thanks to the dopamine hit you get from doing the workout.

6. I set aside time to eat breakfast. I flip flop between eating oats or a cooked breakfast. Having a good breakfast ensures I am fuelling my body and will stop me from grabbing something less nutritious on the go, or being tempted to snack.

The funny thing is, if I stop my morning routine, I can definitely feel the difference. If I go long periods of time without having a morning to reflect and set my intentions, then I am less productive, have less clarity and over a few days get a bit cranky so it's served me well.

Work environment.

Seeing as we spend a lot of time at work, it would make sense to address this environment, so it supports our overall goal. Before I was a Personal Trainer, I actually worked in an office 9-5, Monday to Friday, so I know only too well the types of habits that can be picked up, depending on the office environment.

Every day it was someone's birthday, wedding or baby shower, which meant there was a constant flow of chocolates, cakes and treats and for someone with a sweet tooth, it was extremely hard to resist. Pub lunches, eating at the desks, vending machines, unhealthy canteen foods, it is little wonder women struggle in this environment and that's just if you work in an office. Some professions will be on the road, this can lead to stopping at service stations on a regular basis and grabbing food on the go, potentially making poor food choices. Other women I coach are responsible for client entertaining and part of their job is to wine and dine colleagues to help build relationships for the company they work for. Then, there are those who work night shifts or long shifts and food choices are limited due to location and surroundings. It can be very easy to blame our working environment and conditions for our poor choices, but that's just an excuse to let you off the hook and not take responsibility for your actions. Whatever your occupation, there will always be some barrier or challenge, but it's down to you to take control and make the right choices and find a way to do this differently, so you can keep moving towards your goals. Much like our home environment, we need to set ourselves up for success in our work environment too, because relying on constant sheer willpower throughout the day, will end up in decision fatigue and that never ends well.

Whether you are in an office based job, on the road, entertaining clients or working shifts, you will have fallen into a comfortable routine and picked up some habits, some off which may not be helpful. For example always saying yes to those cakes in the office, even when you are not hungry, or always picking up a chocolate bar from a garage whenever you buy fuel for your car, or having good intensions to have a chicken and pesto salad for lunch, but end up buying a burger and fries instead. I know, because I used to do the same, I used to go through phases of being healthy and then not. One of my unhealthy phases meant every morning I would go to the work canteen and make myself fresh granary toast with butter, then about 10 am go back and buy a giant cookie or two, I wasn't even hungry but it became a daily routine and habit I had fallen into.   Ultimately this unhealthy routine led to some unwanted fat gain, because I wasn't active enough to use those extra cookie calories. The good news is, I disrupted that routine and created myself a new one and that means you can too.

Plan and prepare

The absolute best way to stay on course towards your goal is to be prepared and get yourself organised. I know, tell you something you don't know already. But are you doing it? My guess is probably not! Most people roll their eyes when I tell them to plan and prepare, because deep down, they already know this, the trouble is they just don't want to hear it. The reason for that is because they were hoping I would have a cool strategy that required less effort to share with them, but we all know that usually it is the most obvious and simple solutions that are the most effective.

Top Tips.

1. Make a packed lunch. Very simple and it will take no longer than 10 mins to do. There is absolutely no reason why you couldn't prepare your packed lunch the night before you go to work or get up ten mins early to do this. If you need food inspiration then Pinterest is an excellent source of finding lots of healthy packed lunch ideas.

2. If there are cakes around the office you have two options; Eat the cake and work this into your daily calories and ditch the guilt. Or you can make sure you have brought a tasty alternative snack with you, that you can enjoy and not feel like you are missing out.

3. Do not eat at your desk. Sure, you may be super busy, but you can take 10-20 mins to go eat your

lunch. If you are eating at your desk or eating whilst driving then your mind is focusing on work. That means you are likely going to miss the cues from your stomach to your brain that let you know when you are satisfied and have eaten enough. Also, you won't notice how good your food taste either. This leads to mindless over eating and snacking.

4. If you are eating out, see if you can chose the restaurant which you eat at, or if that decision is out of your hands, then make sure you preview the menu online and decide on what you will have before you go. This does two things; Firstly, you can plan ahead and work the rest of your days' nutrition around the meal. Secondly, it prevents you from making on the spot poor choices.

5. When out and about travelling, either by car or on foot, make sure you keep some healthy 100-200 calorie snacks in your bag, in case you get caught out and feel peckish.

6. These days, most services stations do offer healthy choices. But, knowing what to eat and what constitutes a healthy days' nutrition is what is best going to serve you here. Bread isn't the devil food (unless you are gluten intolerant). A sandwich is a perfectly acceptable option if it fits within your daily calories. It's when you pick up a meal deal, adding in a packet of crisps and a can of fizzy pop, plus that granola bar, which will probably tip you over the edge.

7. Ditch the excuses. Using the excuses "I don't have time" or "I didn't have a choice". This kind of talk is you trying to justify your actions. There is always a choice, so don't let yourself off the hook and check out the menu online. This means you can decide what you are going to eat before even going there

enabling you to plan the rest of your day around the events so you can stay within your calorie goals for the day.

Clean up your environment.

Wherever you work, having a clean working environment will help clear the mind. If your desk, car or workspace is messy and unorganised, how can you have the clarity to make the right choices and feel focused? So, have a little spring clean and notice the difference.

Training environment.

Your training environment, or place where you like to workout also has a lot to do with whether you will be successful or not in staying consistent with your workouts. I have definitely been in different gyms, classes and other fitness environments where I felt either really motivated or just meh. Every gym has a different feel to it and every class has a different energy. Personally, I am not a fan of big commercial gyms, I find them too crowded, too many people, I get annoyed that I can't just crack on with my workout and lose my flow. Whereas, if you put me in a independent and smaller gym, I am in my element, often there are far less people, more sense of community and I'm not waiting and wasting time to use a piece of equipment. Likewise, if I do a fitness class, I'm looking for the ones that make me smile, that make it fun. It basically comes down to enjoyment, so the best advice I can give you is to keep trying different gyms, classes, workouts until you find what clicks for you. But, one thing is for sure, if you don't try, then you will never know. To ensure you stay consistent with your exercise, then you will need to look forward to going, because if your initial though is "urgh, I don't want to go", then after a couple of weeks you will be paying for a gym membership you will never use.

Convenience.

The convenience of your workout is important and can potentially be a big barrier, which stands in the way. There is actually a lot to consider here, such as when, where and how? Let's look at the when first. At what time of day does exercise work for you best? Finding the time to get a workout in can be tricky if you are busy. However, if getting into shape is important to you, then this excuse isn't an option. It's down to you to either create or find time in your day, but you need to make sure it works for you, otherwise you will not be able stick with it. If you have had a long day and you are mentally exhausted, how likely is it that you will have the discipline to get to the gym, workout from home or go for a run? And even if you could do that for a couple of weeks, would you be able to keep that up long term? On the flip side, maybe working out in the evening is just what you need to shake off the stress and feel refreshed? Maybe you are a morning person or you have more time in the morning to exercise. Doing a workout first thing in the morning ensures you tick that box and you can crack on with the rest of your day. I am definitely a morning person personally, I am self aware enough to know that if it doesn't happen in the first half of my day then it may not happen at all. You may need to give yourself a trial, see how you feel on a week of mornings, midday (if possible) or evenings.

Next up is where. So, I already covered the training environment, but I didn't touch on location. The location you are doing your workouts will have an impact on your mentality towards these sessions. If a gym or class is too far away, it may put you off going.

Last of all let's look at how. How are you going to get your workout in? What barriers potentially stand in your way of achieving this? Is it children being demanding, is it your willpower and motivation? This is when organisation works a treat. I get up early every week day morning to do workouts and a trick I picked up was to neatly lay out my workout clothes on the floor next to my bed the night before. This helps me be consistent by removing that choice of what to wear first thing in the morning and also it's a reminder of the promise I made with myself the night before. But, maybe you're going straight after work and if so, keeping your gym bag in the car will mean you can just go without having to take a detour home and lose motivation. If you are a Mum, then carving time out for you is important. Could your partner, friend or family member look after your little angels? Could you plan a workout around their bedtime and exercise from home? Or, why not get them to join in, I tried that once and I can tell you that my enthusiasm for fitness has not rubbed off on my children...yet! But they are watching me and when they are ready, they will have learnt from my example. Is there a crèche at your gym? So what I am getting at here is that for every problem there is always a solution if you look for it. Just by planning ahead and anticipating what potentially might prevent you from your workout, you can get a clear plan of action in place that works for you.

Accountability.

Everyone is different and we all have different motivators, you just need to know what makes you tick. I like to train alone when it comes to weight training, but I have also recently taken up Salsa Dancing, which means I am around lots of people, so these are two very different environments, but I use accountability for both. For my weight training and nutrition, I have a coach and I have a goal and these keep me accountable. If I mess up or miss a check in, then I am letting my Coach down and then, I also have the burden of getting closer to reaching my goal. When it comes to my Salsa dancing, I stay consistent with that because I want to keep improving and dance better (my competitive streak comes into play here). But also, Salsa is a group activity and I don't want to let the others down by not showing up. So what holds you accountable? Is having a goal and a strong why enough and you enjoy working on this alone? Do you need the support of others, in which case maybe having a workout buddy or a attending a class or having a personal trainer is something you need to ensure you keep showing up?

Chapter 15

Healthy habits.

Us humans are creatures of habit. We live blissfully in our comfort zones, based around our daily routines and habits. Our daily routines keep structure to our day and our habits are made up from things we find pleasure in, like having a cup of coffee first thing in the morning or things we must do, like brushing our teeth. Routines and habits serve a purpose, because they provide us with certainty, which our brains love and they helps remove the need to make more decisions. We would have performed habits like drinking coffee and brushing our teeth over and over until they become second nature and easy to do. But, there would have been a time when these habits were new and you had to learn them. Let's go back to when you were a small child and brushing your teeth was a hard task, you would likely have been supervised by mum or dad to make sure you didn't swallow the toothpaste and brushed your teeth properly. But, over time and with practice, brushing your teeth became easy. This is just like any habit and interestingly, some are easier to pick up than others. Going back to brushing your teeth, this habit would have probably taken a while to master, because let's face it, as a child it's pretty boring. How many times were you told to go back up stairs and brush them properly? I know that happened to me a lot. It wasn't till I got a little older, I realised that the benefits were worth having, like having fresh breath and nice teeth. Compare that habit to say having three biscuits after school and I had no problem forming that instantly, because I saw the benefits of this straight away.

Rewards

A habit I had for years was to wake up and make a lovely fresh cup of coffee. It's never a chore, I always looked forward to it and no matter how tired I may have been I was never too tired to make this cup of coffee. The reason why this habit stuck, was because I had plenty of practice, but more importantly the feel good factor "reward" I got from having my morning coffee, further drove me to continue and reinforced this behaviour. You don't find many people carrying on a habit that they do not enjoy, or it doesn't offer some kind of reward. The feel good sensation we experience is called dopamine, one of our happy hormones and that's why habits can be really hard to change. People have tried to define the number of days it takes to learn a new habit, various numbers like 21 days or 60 days have been thrown around but I don't believe in this. For me I have stopped some habits that I could never go back to like smoking for instance, yes I used to smoke. Then, there are other habits like eating chocolate which will always be there, because I still enjoy it and in this case it's being more self aware about my actions and clear about my goals, that allows me to manage this habit in a healthy manner.

Here is how I see habits. Imagine there is a meadow with tall grass and flowers and you can see a clear pathway through the grass and on the ground where people have walked over and over again. Now, imagine that people decided to change route and found another way to the river and started to walk the new route every day. What do you think would happen? This new pathway would become clearer as the grass would give way. However, the old pathway would still be there, but now because nobody uses this, it's become overgrown with grass again. You can still access the river using the old pathway and if you changed routes again it would become clearer.

That analogy is exactly how habits work. The more we do something, the stronger that habit becomes. The less we do it, the weaker the habit is and it will fade but never really goes. The only time a habit will stop entirely and you will never go back to it, is if there is no longer a reward to the outcome. This is why I no longer enjoy smoking, because the reward doesn't serve me, I don't enjoy it, I feel sick, I don't like smelling of smoke and it's no good for my health. It's also why I still enjoy chocolate because I do enjoy that reward, which basically comes down to the taste. So knowing that habits are reinforced by a feel good factor, it would be pointless trying to create a new habit around something you didn't enjoy.

If you have a whole bunch of unhealthy habits you are looking to change, it would be a great idea to focus on changing just one thing at a time. Trust me, if you try and change everything all at once, you will be heading for overwhelm. Remember our brains like certainty and keeping the decision making to a minimum, so if you asking your brain to get on board whilst you switch up everything, you may struggle to stick to it and end up throwing the towel in. Remember, when we are overwhelmed or stressed, our clever brains step up to and find the quickest way back to certainty and that is usually found in the comfort of our old habits. We have all been there and it's normal, you shouldn't consider this a failure just a learning curve. The best thing to do is to dust yourself down and try again. It takes times to build new habits and you must expect some blips along the way.

A useful tip when it comes to changing habits would be to start with something small. Identify a habit which doesn't serve you well, but instead of completely removing it, simply make a swap for another habit which is a healthier alternative and helps you move the needle closer towards your goal. Here are a couple of examples of how you could make healthier alternative swaps.

Scenario 1: You love your daily trip to the coffee shop and always have a large latte with two sugars. Instead of stopping doing something you enjoy all together, you simply swap your regular latte for skinny latte and sweetener instead. This is a less calorific option and you still get the same feel good sensation, your dopamine hit, and you haven't had to change too much to achieve this. This small step will save you around 100 calories a day which add up to 700 in a week! That's pretty epic.

Scenario 2: After a long day, you finally sit down and enjoy your favourite chocolate bar, which is around about 250 calories. Well, how about swapping this for a healthier choice of a small bag of sweet popcorn, or two squares of dark chocolate, or some fruit, or two Jaffa cakes, anything sweet that would be less calorific that you may enjoy. Again saving you 100 calories a day.

As you can see, these seemly small healthier swaps can add up to some big changes and it's much more manageable to replace one habit with another healthier alternative, as long as it offers the same reward and feel good factor in the end.

Chapter 16

People and influences.

I wanted to touch on how the people we surround ourselves with can affect and even influence our behaviours and mind set, sometimes for the better and sometime for the worse. There is a saying, which goes something like this "You are the sum of the five people you spend the most time with". When I first heard this, it really made me think of the different phases of my life I have been through, the different kinds of company I kept and it's true, I shared similarities to those I spent the most time with. You will probably find the same. These days I am careful who I spend time with, because I understand the impact the right or wrong people around you can have. The right people can lift you, inspire you, grow with you and have very positive impacts, but the wrong people can hold you back or worse still pull you down.

Getting fitter and healthier will require some lifestyle

changes and that could mean some social changes may need to happen as well. I am not saying you need to un-friend everybody in your social circle that eats cake. But, I am saying you should look to introduce a couple of people into your circle who share common goals and interests, because they will have a positive influence and help you move closer to where you want to be. It can be very hard to make change when you are doing it on your own, but it's much easier when you have a team of up lifting people on board.

Push back and Resistance

As the saying goes, *"Everybody wants you to do good, but never better than them." Unknown.*

Don't expect everyone to be cheering you on. I say this, because there will inevitably be a time when someone will express their unwanted opinion and make comments about what you are doing. I experienced some negativity from various people in the past and from talking to other women. I know many have gone through the same, it seems to be pretty common. After I hired my Personal Trainer, I started to get serious about fitness, that's when the push back and resistance started, not off many just one or two people that couldn't understand what I was doing or even why, but what was hard was this resistance was coming from my husband.

I would always look forward to my gym sessions and loved

it even more when I started seeing results. However, my husband didn't love it, well at least to start with anyway. Often, when I was just about to leave the house and head to the gym for a workout, he would say things like "Going to the gym again?" or "Don't end up looking like a man", sometimes he would roll his eyes in contempt. As soon as he said or did things like this, my mood shifted and I would go from feeling super pumped up and ready to go, to then feeling like I was doing something wrong and being selfish, like I was neglecting my family. Luckily for me, I am stubborn and went anyway. Other times, I would be teased by work colleagues or friends and have comments made like "Don't get too skinny" or "You eating that rabbit food again?" Whilst these may seem like harmless comments and they were only joking around, it can wear you down and be upsetting if people keep chipping away at you.

What you need to know is that these people are not intentionally being gits. Think of this more of a knee jerk reaction to their feelings. Here is what's actually going on. Your change in lifestyle, body and mind set is stirring emotions in other people. For some people that emotion maybe jealousy, they see you doing something they wish they could do, but haven't yet been able to achieve. It could be uncertainty, this is common in partners because they feel threatened as you improve how you look and gain confidence, it changes the dynamics of a relationship. Ultimately, this is other people projecting their fears and insecurities onto you and it absolutely isn't your fault. People fear change, as it brings the unknown, but give it time and eventually they will come round as you create a new normal; a fitter and healthier normal. In the meantime, don't worry about what anyone else thinks.

Chapter 17

Sleep

Sleep is a basic human need just like food and water, without sleep we are not able to function at our best. Sleep deprivation and tiredness can trigger some interesting body responses, which definitely won't help you reach your fat loss goal. I work with a lot of women who are either not getting enough sleep, or the quality of sleep is very poor and this can be for a number of reasons. What I have found is, that when we take things back to basics, their sleep dramatically improves. It's said that an adult needs on average seven hours sleep per night, however some people function perfectly fine on less, whilst others may need more. Without adequate sleep, the body can be reluctant to cooperate with your goals in the pursuit of fat loss, or performing at it's best and this is due to the stress that a lack of sleep places on the body. So, if you are struggling with sleep, then keep reading, as I will go into what common mistakes people make and how to get round these.

Circadian Clock

Our bodies are governed by a biological clock otherwise known as the Circadian clock. Throughout the day, the body will undergo different changes in hormones, body temperatures, cortisol levels and blood pressure all based on the Circadian clock. The Circadian Clock is the natural flow our bodies follow and if we go against the Circadian clock, we can feel pretty rubbish. Ever noticed how refreshed you feel when you to wake up naturally with the sun rise, rather than the sudden shock of the alarm clock? It's no coincidence. As the sunrises, our body will go through a series of biological changes that gently wakes us up from sleep, our blood pressure starts to rise, cortisol levels increase (our stress hormone) and the secretion of melatonin (sleep hormone) ceases, all gearing us to wake up. Likewise, as the sun sets our body temperature rises, our cortisol levels drop and melatonin secretions start readying us for sleep.

The effects of inadequate or lack of sleep

So what happens to the body when sleep isn't as it should be? Well, the reason I am bringing up the topic of sleep, is because it does have a correlation to someone's ability to lose fat.

1. An obvious effect would be the sensation of feeling tired and having a lack of energy, but if you have a number nights of poor quality sleep, babies are really good at disrupting sleep, then fatigue and a lack of motivation can also set in.
2. If you have ever had a bad nights' sleep, you will know only too well how snappy this can make you. So mood swings can be expected.

3. Your mental skills and co-ordination can be affected, you're less likely to be as sharp and on the ball as you would be and clumsy.

4. You won't be able to cope with stress as well.

5. You may find your immune system will take a battering. You're more susceptible to picking up colds and infections.

6. You may gain weight due to sugar cravings to boost your energy due to feeling tired.

So, now you know why sleep is so important to you, it's time to make some changes in order to reap the benefits of it.

Caffeine

I think we all know that caffeine is a stimulant, so it seems like an obvious place to start would be to look at your caffeine intake. Did you know that when you drink a cup of coffee it's takes around 45 mins for it to be absorbed and approximately half of that caffeine will still be in your system five hours later? As I have gotten older, my tolerance to caffeine has definitely gotten less and I find myself tired yet laying in bed unable to switch my brain off. If this has ever happened to you, then you will understand how frustrating it is to desperately want to sleep, but instead you're just laid there thinking about all sorts of randomness. Such an episode happened a few years ago and it wasn't until the next day, I suddenly had a light bulb moment and realised why. That afternoon I had consumed a kick ass energy drink about 4pm prior to my gym session, I did my gym session as normal, then went to bed at 10pm, but sleep wasn't happening. So I learnt a lesson there. Seeing as caffeine is a stimulant, it would be wise to not drink coffee past 4pm as this is when our cortisol levels naturally drop and drinking caffeine, it will raise cortisol levels again, which is not ideal. I take this one step further and don't drink caffeine beyond the first half of my day.

Get a routine.

I have probably mentioned once or twice that us Humans love a good routine and when it comes to our bedtimes it's no different. You can train yourself to stay awake late or go to bed early. I get up pretty early during the week usually 5am or 5.30am, so to make sure I get enough sleep, I reversed engineered my bedtime on getting my seven hours sleep, which meant my bedtime would need to be around 10pm. I would recommend you look at your own bedtime and see if you can work out your perfect bedtime, so you can wake up feeling refreshed. Once you have, it will likely take a week to establish a routine, as to start with you may not feel tired.

Unplug

This is a difficult one for people to do, to detach from technology and let our brains have a rest. I shall confess, as I am the worst for this, I work online so I'm always answering emails, on social media and then, I will be found chilling out on the sofa with another huge screen in front of me. But, I do force myself to take breaks now and then, but I also practice a strict no screen routine before bedtime. These days, we are never more than arms reach away from our mobiles and let's not forget TVs, Laptops and

Tablets. But, did you know that these screens are throwing off what is called blue light and it is this blue light that disrupts the production of melatonin. Melatonin is the hormone that helps us sleep and around 9pm our melatonin levels rise sharply in the blood making us feel tired. If you are using screens before bed, then you will be exposed to blue light whilst also stimulating your mind, which is the complete opposite of what you should be doing, because in the evenings we ideally want to be winding down.

TOP TIP: To help your brain switch off and to allow Melatonin secretion, try and put all screens down and do something relaxing in the 30 mins before you go to bed. Something like stretching, reading a book, having a bath or anything like that.

Brain dump.

This is one of my favourites. Like most women I rarely switch off, we have so much going on in our heads, ideas floating around, a never ending to do list, and things I need to remember. If I attempt to go to bed without doing a brain dump there is no chance of me relaxing properly, because I will be thinking of everything I need to do tomorrow. So here's what I do to combat this. Before I go to bed, I write down everything I have to do on my to do list for the next day, so I know I won't forget, enabling me to drift off to sleep peacefully knowing that it's all out of my head and written down, which makes space in my brain. Another thing I like to do is keep a note pad and pen by my bedside table, so if a random through pops up, then I can jot it down and know it will be there in the morning when I wake up.

Sleeping environment.

Our bedrooms should be used for two things and that is sleeping and sex. We absolutely shouldn't be doing work from bed, watching TV or playing on our phones, because our brains will start to make associations with these actions to our rooms and instead of the bedroom being a relaxing place, it becomes just like any other room in the house.

Does your bedroom have technology everywhere? Mobile phone docking stations, flashing radio clocks and TV? If so, then it's likely that the lights, which are coming from these devices, are affecting your sleep. Your phone flashing at every notification or message, the TV light preventing melatonin secretion, maybe streetlights are coming through the window? Ideally your room should be in complete darkness.

I am a big fan of white noise, white noise is a continuous low level back ground noise that's help you to relax. I sleep with a fan going which serves two purposes helping me keep cool at night, whilst being that low level back ground noise as well. However, some people may prefer complete silence. Room temperature is also really important, too hot or too cold and you will have an uncomfortable sleep.

Other considerations to watch out for are ...

Alcohol before bed, a common sleep disruptor is alcohol. People who drink will find that the initial going to sleep isn't a problem as it can aid drifting off, but it does disrupt the deep sleep cycle, leaving us feeling tired and groggy the next day. Also drinking too much liquid before bed will increase the likelihood for the need to go to the toilet during the night.

Part 4. Exercise and Activity

If fat loss, building muscle, losing weight or increasing your fitness abilities are the goal, then you are going to need to incorporate some movement and exercise into your day to help make this happen. A fact worth remembering is that the majority of your fat loss results will come as a result of being in a calories deficit through your nutrition, around 70% approximately for the average women. The exception to that rule would be anyone who partakes in activities like running marathons or doing other endurance sports that burn a lot of energy and if that's the case your nutrition needs to support your training. But, for the sake of this book, let's say you are looking to lose body fat, tone up and improve overall fitness. In this section, I am going to touch on why women should perform some sort of resistance training, why doing too much exercise could be hindering your progress and why I recommend getting your N.E.A.T on. You may have expected that this section would be a lot longer, the trick is to keeping it simple. People make this far too complicated and it doesn't need to be.

Chapter 18

Why women should do resistance training

Resistance training can come in many forms such as weight training, HIIT workouts, bodyweight resistance training, spin classes, body pump classes, boxing and many more, really anything that applies a resistance against the muscle. There are so many benefits to resistance training and as we age, it become more important that we incorporate some form of resistance training into our exercise regime.

It's no secret that I am a big fan of weight training. When I first started weight training all those years ago, I remember feeling nervous and the thought of going into the free weights area seemed a little intimidating with all the grunting men and their huge muscles. I was so worried about what people were thinking about me, that I made it out to be far worse in my head than it actually turned out to be in reality. I know that lots of women worry about the same thing, the fear of judgement can be crippling, so I have a lot of empathy for women new to the gym environment and can relate to that daunting feeling. If stepping into the gym is a worry of yours, my advice would be give it two weeks. After two weeks, that worry will have melted away, as you would of gained more confidence and become more familiar with your surroundings and the exercises. Had I let the fear get to me and not taken that first step, then things would look very different for me right now. I wouldn't have grown in confidence, I wouldn't be a Personal Trainer, this book would never have happened and that would have all been because I made that decision to let the fear of judgment stop me. I am happy to say that I didn't and you shouldn't either. If you are worried, then why not see if a friend will come with you a few times or a gym instructor can show you a few exercises.

Benefits of Resistance Training

Everyone should be performing some sort of resistance training and it doesn't have to be gym based either. As long as you're placing force through the muscles, then that is still a form of resistance training. But, the question is why? Why should you incorporate resistance training into your weekly regime? Here are a few reasons below:-

- Resistance training will increase muscle mass and this in turn will make you a more efficient fat burning machine, sounds pretty cool doesn't it. The reason for this is, the more muscle mass a person has, the more energy their body uses at rest to simply maintain the muscle. This is good news for you, as it means your daily calorie threshold increases due to your body being able to handle slightly more calories than before without gaining excess fat. And who doesn't love more food?
- Another great benefit of resistance training is, it keeps us strong by building muscle, which supports our joints and protects our spine from injury.
- Resistance training can help with improving posture. If you have any imbalances such as slouching forwards and rounding of the

shoulders, then resistance training and focusing on the back can help pull the shoulders back to correct this and improve your posture.

- Resistance training helps to maintain muscle mass and slows down the process of muscle wastage as we get older, which occurs in women from around the ages of 35 and this speeds up as we enter menopause.

- Resistance training helps to build bone density and prevents osteoporosis, brittle bones disease, making you less likely to suffer with fractures and breaks as you age. Again, the risk increase as we enter menopause.

- Body composition will change. The great thing about resistance training and building muscle is you can create more shape to your body. A perkier rounder bottom, shapely firm legs, toned upper arms and tighter looking tummy.

- The workouts are a lot more interesting and offer more variation. Nobody wants to run on a treadmill for 60 mins, when you could be doing a far more interesting workout.

As you can see, there are a lot of benefits to resistance training and some with significant health benefits too. As we age, including some sort of resistance training into our exercise regime becomes even more important to ensure we stay strong and able bodied.

Chapter 19

Are you doing too much exercise?

Oh boy, I was guilty of this in the past and I know many women probably fall into this trap of doing to much exercise without even realising it. But, we can be forgiven for making this mistake, as logic would suggest that the more you exercise, the more calories you burn, so why would you not do as much as possible, it seems like a no brainer! Doing too much exercise or not having enough time to recover from physical activity can and will hinder your progress, making it harder to see results. But, the reality of doing too much physical activity and not having enough recovery time, means that you are stressing out the body and putting yourself at risk of injury or burn out. In this case, more doesn't always mean better.

Back in the day, I was a workout junkie before I knew any better and here is what happened to me. After qualifying as a Personal Trainer I set up a local Bootcamp which was just for women. This Bootcamp was three evenings a week and it was a High Intensity class which lasted a full 60 mins. It was hard, it was intense and we loved it because you would leave my Bootcamp dripping with sweat. Within a month, the Bootcamp was so popular, I had to add another class to accommodate the demand. This meant I was now doing back to back Bootcamp sessions as well as my usual five days weight training and an extra bonus Bootcamp on a Saturday. So it's safe to say, I was definitely doing enough exercise, in a week it worked out that I was doing a total of 12 hours high intensity training. I look at this now and wonder how on earth I kept going like this for so long, two years to be exact. Frustratingly, however, I never seemed to lose the fat, I was doing so much exercise and burning a ton of calories, but the fat just wasn't shifting! You would have thought I'd have been a lean machine but I wasn't and sat comfortably at a size 12 and had plenty of excess fat stored around my hips, bum, upper thighs and backs of my arms and no matter how much I tried, it just didn't go.

There are two reasons for this. I was training like an athlete, but I wasn't fuelling my body like an athlete, or giving myself enough rest. I was desperate to see results, so I put myself into huge calories deficit and ate between 900-1200 calories a day, which wasn't enough to support my body under normal circumstances, let alone the amount of exercise I was doing. By dramatically under eating and under recovering, I was placing my body under a lot of physical stress. As you know from the chapter on stress earlier, you will remember I mentioned that stress causes our body to store fat, especially around the tummy area, that was exactly the issue I was having. This wasn't the only problem I had, because I was so restrictive with my calories during the week, what do you think happened at the weekend? That's right, I binged on anything carby and fatty, because my body was crying out for energy. This became a really unhealthy weekend habit that I developed and even justified it by calling it a "cheat meal", but in my case the cheat meal turned into a day, which turned into the entire weekend. This unhealthy habit meant that, whilst I was in a calories deficit all week, the weekend binges cancelled any progress I had made, taking my body out of a calories deficit and into a calorie surplus, meaning I gained fat instead losing it. Not eating enough and giving our bodies enough recovery time is something I see a lot of women do. I have seen women train for marathons who don't understand the importance of fuelling their body correctly. Typically, what happens with women that run long distances and under eat is, they experience muscle wastage, they will find their body will hold on to fat stores whilst it uses muscle for fuel instead, which is not ideal.

After a couple of years of this and getting nowhere, I decided that I must be doing something wrong and reached out to a fellow PT friend of mine called Dan Mitchell. This time, my choice of Personal Trainer was based on results and trusting his methods, unlike before. I asked Dan to help me get lean and prep me for a Bikini Fitness Competition and luckily he obliged. The very first thing he did was up my calorie intake and he bumped me up to 1900 calories a day. Then, he told me to take down my activity level to help reduce the stress to my body, so that put a stop to me joining in with my Bootcamp sessions and I did just four weight training sessions a week. Just to clarify, this meant I went from 12 hours a week right down to four hours of just resistance training a week. This approach seemed alien to me, but I trusted Dan and did exactly as he said. The only other activity I did was to look at my N.E.A.T, and kept a check on my daily step count. I shall go more into N.E.A.T in another chapter.

The results were astonishing. Immediately, my body responded and I looked leaner in just a week, this was my body thanking me for not stressing it out. I dropped the water retention and inflammation and that alone made a huge difference. I developed a better relationship with food, because I wasn't being so restrictive and therefore I wasn't binging on the weekends either. A few more weeks in and you could see my body shape changing, my tummy and hips gradually co-operating and losing fat from these areas too which was a miracle in itself. In just 12 weeks, I had gone from a size 12 to a size 8 and achieved the leanest, strongest and least stressed version of myself ever. I stood on stage and won 1st place in my Bikini Fitness Competition. It was by going through this process, I finally understood the impact that the physical stress had on my body. Once I gave my body what it needed, my body was then able to give me what I wanted. Ever since then, it has been something I have been helping women understand and achieve through my coaching programs.

Here are two really useful tips to help you avoid falling into this trap.

1. Make sure you have 2-3 rest days each week. This means backing off from your main training, whether that's weight training or running and allow the body to repair and recover properly. You can add in some active recovery like yoga or walking which will give you those endorphins you crave without stressing out the body. This is called active recovery.

2. Fuel your body properly. If you are performing high intensity exercise or taking part in endurance sports, then ensure you are giving your body the fuel it needs to support your training. This will prevent muscle wastage, help to reduce stress by increasing calories and get more nutrients into

the body. It will also prevent you from binging on foods due to being too restrictive.

Chapter 20

N.E.A.T

What is N.E.A.T? Well it's really neat actually (sorry bad pun). N.E.A.T is really effective and it's usually overlooked as a key tool in the fat loss game. N.E.A.T Stands for Non Exercise Activity Thermogenesis, which is a fancy way of saying activity that isn't classed as exercise. Think walking, fidgeting, standing and moving the body around. Here is an interesting fact. When it comes to fat loss 70% of this will come down to your nutrition, 5% will be down to your workout in the gym and 25% of it will be down to your daily activity, aka your N.E.A.T. Something to think about.....

N.E.A.T doesn't negate the importance of exercise. Exercise has long term advantages, for example building cardiovascular health and muscle. But, your overall activity will go a long way to support your fat loss goals without stressing out the body by adding in extra grueling workouts or spending forever on a piece of cardio equipment. I don't know about you, but the idea of being on a treadmill staring at one spot for hours is not appealing and to do that continuously, week in week out, makes me want to cry. I've been there and done that. Never again!

In today's world, we are far more sedentary than we were 20, 50 and 100 years ago. Unless you have an active job or are on your feet all day, most people find themselves sat down for large portions of their day. We wake up, go to work either by car, train or bus, then at work we sit down at a desk for eight hours, go home, sit down for dinner and again sit down in front of the telly to keep us company as we scroll through social media. (does anyone else do that or is it just me?). If you wear a step tracker or smart watch, then you will see that you may clock up as little as 2-3,000 steps a day. The recommended is 10,000 steps. If you are active and spend a lot of your day on your feet, then that is going to help keep your N.E.A.T up.

So how do you increase your daily activity? First of all, we need to remember this is a lifestyle change and not a race, so if you are doing 3,000 steps a day, is it sustainable for you to suddenly up this to 10,000? It might be better to increase a couple of thousand steps every month to help you gradually get used to a more active lifestyle. Things you can do to help you up your daily activity are:-

- Park the car further away and walk more
- Take the stairs instead of the lift
- Make sure you get up every hour and move around
- Take your dog on longer walks or if you don't have a dog just get your trainers on and get outside.
- Take the kids to the park and join in the fun
- Housework, I like this idea because I hate house work, but if I think about how much moving I do it does help.

- Go for family walks at the weekend or do fun things that mean you're not sitting down.

At the start of your fat loss journey, just by adding in regular exercise sessions, it will be enough to see results. But, as the weeks go by and your body adapts, you will need to tweak things like upping activity levels or lowering calories slightly to keep progressing or else your body will plateau. I would recommend getting yourself a step counter of some description and these can vary in price, I have had expensive smart watches that's do all kinds of fancy thing like track your heart rate, currently I use a basic pedometer that I wear on my wrist which I bough online for £20.

The End

And Ta'da, that's it, you have reached the end of this book. Thank you for taking the time to read this and trusting in me to guide you back to basics. This books' purpose was to help sift through all the fluff, the nonsense, the gimmicks and the myths around fat loss and give you the fundamental principles of what it really takes to be successful in your body goals. You can be safe in the knowledge that by covering the basics consistently you will make progress. It's my mission to help women take control of their health and fitness through the power of movement, nutrition and mindset before looking for external solutions.

"You already have everything you need to be successful, you just need to believe in yourself a little more" Vanessa French

I truly believe that the possibilities of what you can achieve are endless. You are capable of achieving a better body, a better mind set and a better relationship with food. You are in the driving seat of your life and in charge of what happens from here. To ensure you get the most out of this book, you may need to read it again or go back to parts and chapters you feel you need to focus on more.

Here are some wise words to leave you with. Change is often hard at first, messy in the middle and beautiful in the end. So keep going, it will be worth it.

Vanessa x

My gifts to you

I wrote this book to give women the truth about what it takes to see results. I really want you to succeed and become leaner, fitter and more confident and to help you achieve this I have created the V.Fit 7 workout sheet. The V.Fit 7 is a worksheet for you to download and use to map out where you go from here and put a plan of action into place. Create your goals, discover your why, practice mindfulness and set yourself up for success. To claim your V.Fit 7 worksheet, simply join my free Facebook community.

https://www.facebook.com/groups/vfitcommunity/

Your next gift is claiming 20% off my six month online coaching program, Project Badass. A six month transformation program, that combines weight training, nutrition and mind set to achieve amazing results. To claim this, type this URL into your browser and fill out the form.

http://eepurl.com/gblauT

Reach out to me

If you have any questions, would like more information or even if you just want to say hi, then make sure you do, I love chatting with you guys. You can find me on social media.

www.vanessafrenchfitness.com My website

Instagram: www.instagram.com/vanessafrenchfitness

Facebook: www.facebook.com/vanessafrenchfitness

Acknowledgements

There are so many people who I would like to say thanks to, because it takes a village and it certainly has taken a village to shape the person who I am today. All the people who impacted my life, taught me lessons, guided me, listened, reached out, I thank you all.

First of all I want to say thank you to my Husband, Jason. I thank you for being the complete opposite of me and having my back. Your unwavering support and belief in me is truly amazing. You are amazing. Thank you to my first born, Jessica. You gave me purpose to my life when I was lost and the drive to change my life for the better. I wanted to show you that history doesn't have to repeat itself and that you can be or do anything if you put the work in. Thank you to my youngest daughter Samantha. It was you who encouraged me to write a book, not this book but that one is coming, I don't think I would have done it unless you gave me that nudge, you are wise beyond your years young lady. Thank you to Dan Mitchell for being a truly awesome coach, you took me under your wing and taught me so much, plus we won a few trophies together in my fitness competitions. Thank you to all my V.Fit and Project Badass members, clients old and new, you guys rock. There are many others I would like to thank, but we would be here all day. Finally a special thank you to my Dad, Eric for being the biggest dreamer I knew and passing that gift down to me.

Special thanks to Wayne Kahn from Studio 1314, for his awesome photography skills and creating such a beautiful photo for the books cover. for allowing me to use front cover.

www.studio1314.co.uk

Vanessa   x

Printed in Great Britain
by Amazon